THE SECRETS OF HOUSEHOLD TOXINS

A Comprehensive Guide to Creating a Non-Toxic Home, Detoxing from Harmful Chemicals, Enhancing Your Health, and Embracing Healthy Living

TAHIRA ISMAIL

Copyright © 2023 by Tahira Ismail - All rights reserved.

No part of this publication may be reproduced, stored, or transmitted in any form or by any means, electronic, mechanical, photocopying, recording, scanning, or otherwise, without written permission from the publisher. It is illegal to copy this book, post it to a website, or distribute it by any other means without permission.

Tahira Ismail asserts the moral right to be identified as the author of this work. Tahira Ismail has no responsibility for the persistence or accuracy of URLs for external or third-party Internet Websites referred to in this publication and does not guarantee that any content on such websites is, or will remain, accurate or appropriate.

Designations used by companies to distinguish their products are often claimed as trademarks. All brand names and product names used in this book and on its cover are trade names, service marks, trademarks, and registered trademarks of their respective owners. The publishers and the book are not associated with any product or vendor mentioned in this book. None of the companies referenced within the book have endorsed the book.

Disclaimer Notice: Please note the information contained within this document is for educational purposes only. All effort has been executed to present accurate, up-to-date, and reliable, complete information. No warranties of any kind are declared or implied. Readers acknowledge that the author is not engaging in the rendering of legal, financial, medical, or professional advice. The content within this book has been derived from various sources. Please consult a licensed professional before attempting any techniques outlined in this book.

By reading this document, the reader agrees that under no circumstances is the author responsible for any losses, direct or indirect, which are incurred as a result of the use of the information contained within this document, including, but not limited to, — errors, omissions, or inaccuracies.

First edition

This book is dedicated to my dear dad for his never-ending encouragement and support, to my husband for being a driving force for me to reach my potential, and to my children, who are a source of endless inspiration.

CONTENTS

Introduction	7
Part I INVISIBLE DANGER	
1. Understanding Toxins & Toxicity	13
2. Processing Toxins	31
Part II THE ACTION PLAN	
3. Detox: The Kitchen and Dining Room	47
4. Detox: The Bathroom & Laundry Room	63
5. Detox: The Bedroom & Office	83
6. Detox: The Living Room & Playroom	95
7. Detox: Basement, Garage, & Outdoors	109
Part III TAKING CONTROL	
8. Making Changes	129
Conclusion	143
Bonus Chapter: DIY Recipes	147
Appendix 1: Glossary	165
Appendix 2: Replacement List	167
Appendix 3: Shopping for Detox Items	169
Appendix 4: Detox Checklist	173
References	175

INTRODUCTION

Sixteen years ago, my two-year-old daughter Zaynab was prescribed steroids. At the time, I didn't think much of it; she had eczema, and it needed to be treated. Steroids were the standard prescription, and my baby was not going to suffer unnecessarily.

A few hours later, I found myself at the local pharmacy picking up the prescription. As I walked out of the building, I took the container out of the paper bag and flipped over the bottle to skim-read the side effects, stopping suddenly as I read *May cause excess hair growth.*

That was shocking—and undesirable. I had been blessed with an abundance of hair and had passed that gene along to my daughter. One thing she did not need was more of it. At that moment, I began my journey into toxin-free living; perhaps it was more based on vanity, but over the next few weeks, I plunged into the world of clean and healthy living. The more I researched, the more I knew I needed to switch to natural

INTRODUCTION

cleaners and soaps, just to start. I did, and my daughter's eczema went away.

As it turns out, in the average home, every room is filled with toxic chemicals and substances. Toilet bowl cleaner. Make-up. Packaged food. Paint. Clothing. Mold. Pesticides. Animal poisons. The list goes on and on. Some items are obviously dangerous as they contain warning signs that they should not be ingested. However, while we don't intentionally swallow them, we still ingest them when we breathe in their fumes, and our skin — the largest organ in our body — absorbs the odors and fumes they release. Like the grocery store cleaning aisle, sometimes we can smell certain ingredients, but more often than not, we can't see, taste, or smell toxins, chemicals, and other pollutants. They can be airborne, on surfaces, or are included in the components of many common household items.

What happened to *you* that triggered your health and wellness journey? Many people are happy to eat clean and healthy most of the time; however, going all the way to ensure that your home is a healthy sanctuary is an area most people tend to avoid. Is it your health? Do you have long-term unexplained chronic illnesses? Are you tired of using products mainstream media and healthcare advocates as 'safe'? When I began this journey, I was unaware of the side effects toxins were having on my body and how they were harming my family. But throughout the process of detoxification, my home became safe, and our bodies healed.

Detoxifying your home is critical to your health and long-term well-being. Unfortunately, many people today don't realize the side effects of the toxicity levels of many household items. While detoxifying your body through juices, teas, and cleanses

INTRODUCTION

can have a drastic positive impact on your body, when you detox your home, the changes will be less drastic immediately. However, you will notice a direct difference: fewer headaches, scarcer rashes, and no burning sensations in your throat or lungs. However, there are even more significant long-term positive results: lower risk of cancer, chronic fatigue diminishing, weight loss, and disappearing allergies. Reducing toxins, especially those known as forever chemicals, can begin to improve your thyroid, liver, and hormones. Your home deserves to be healthy. You need to do this for yourself and your family. As they say, if you treat it well, it will treat you well.

When I first began my home detoxing journey, I wanted to do it all in one day. However, I quickly learned that all good things resulting in lasting changes must be understood first and then built up and repeated. It is like a couch potato wanting to run a marathon: on their first day of training, they don't run the entire 26.2 miles in one go. To learn how to run a marathon, you need a trainer — someone who will teach you how to stretch, what to eat, and by what methods you can build your endurance. Your home detoxifying journey will be just like that. Together we will begin with the basics: learning what toxins are, where they are found in the home, and how to identify them. From there, we can tackle your home one room at a time. We are not looking for quick fixes that cause us to crash and burn just as fast as we started; rather, we are in this together for the long haul. Step by step, we will walk towards having a pure, toxin-free home together. My goal is that one year from today, you stop and look back at how far you have come and realize that you are never returning to that harmful lifestyle.

From eliminating materials with toxic chemicals to purifying the air with healthy and aesthetic plants, this book will trans-

INTRODUCTION

form your home and your life. We will evaluate various cleaning products and understand what is safe versus what is harmful. We will also discuss which toxins to avoid, which ones to minimize, and which ones we can substitute for healthier alternatives. Say goodbye to common chemical pollutants and hello to friendlier eco alternatives.

Today, my home is well into its detoxification journey. While I sometimes wish that I had known the side effects of using different types of toxins much earlier, I don't look back on those years in shame or disgust: I was doing the best I could with the knowledge I had. However, going forward, the choices I make will be for my family's health and safety — and I wish the same for your family. It is time to make our homes fresh, clean, and safe, but in a responsible manner. So, let's get started on detoxifying your home!

PART I

INVISIBLE DANGER

1

UNDERSTANDING TOXINS & TOXICITY

> *"Household exposure studies, including those conducted by Silent Spring Institute, show that people are exposed to complex mixtures of indoor toxics from building materials and a myriad of consumer products. Pollutants in homes are likely to have multiple health effects because many are classified as endocrine disrupting compounds (EDCs), with the ability to interfere with the body's hormone system."*
>
> — SARAH DUNAGAN[1]

In 2020, of the top sixty-five toxic chemicals found in homes, more than 5,000 tons of these were released throughout California households. The source? Everyday household consumer products such as cleaners, disinfectants, detergents, cosmetics, and the like.

Before we dive into the effects toxins have on our bodies, we must first examine what toxins are and why they are dangerous for our health. This includes the most common household toxins (along with a few that are often found in the workplace). The names of these toxins may sound familiar to you, but an in-depth understanding of what they are and some of their side effects is required to create a lasting change in your home.

WHAT IS A TOXIN?

A toxin is a natural substance (such as a bacteria or germ) produced by plants or animals that can cause harm or permanent damage to the body — and, in extreme cases, can be fatal. Toxins can be airborne, on surfaces, or in solid form, and when they come into contact with people through inhalation, skin absorption, or digestion, they can wreak havoc on nearly every part of the body. A minuscule particle not visible to the naked eye can cause more damage to a body than most people realize. Toxins can be divided into six broad categories:

1. Genitotoxins – toxins that damage reproductive organs (fallopian tubes, ovaries, uterus, testicles, etc.) and urinary organs (kidneys, bladder, prostate, urethra, etc.).
2. Hemotoxins – toxins that damage, destroy, or mutilate red blood cells and negatively affect red blood cells' clotting abilities.
3. Hepatotoxins – toxins that damage the liver.
4. Necrotoxins – toxins that destroy or damage cells.
5. Neurotoxins – toxins that negatively impact the nervous system by damaging nerve tissues (found in and used in the brain and spinal cord).
6. Phototoxins – toxins that cause allergic reactions on the skin for some people (common phototoxins include marigolds; St. John's Wort; some essential oils, herbs,

and perfumes; and umbelliferous plants such as celery, carrots, and parsley.)

Certain animals, such as bees, jellyfish, and rattlesnakes, and plants, such as agaric mushrooms, are well known to be toxic to humans, and therefore we do our best to avoid them. In some cases, contact with a particular animal toxin can cause death, whereas at other times, they affect your health, either short-term or long-term. As this book deals primarily with detoxing your home, we will assume that you don't keep poisonous animals in your home as pets and will end the discussion of toxic animals here!

Toxins are frequently found in household products to make them more effective and durable, or as a cheap alternative to safe quality products. Some medications use toxins in tiny doses to treat an ailment, whereas, in large amounts, they would be poisonous or lethal. Certain metals and natural chemical compounds are also toxic to the human body. Overall, toxins are dangerous for your health, environment, safety, and property.

Several years ago, I was visiting my parents with my son when the house cleaner arrived. I didn't think much of it initially, but as a few hours passed, my son and I noticed that we were getting headaches. By this point, I had been using natural cleaners in my own home for several years and had practically forgotten the reactions chemicals could cause. Realizing something needed to be done, I spoke to the housecleaner, who was more than willing to switch to natural cleaners so long as I purchased the initial set so that she knew going forward what to buy.

One dangerous aspect of toxins is that many of them are unnoticeable through taste, touch, or scent. When toxins begin to build up in your body, over time, you will start to feel sluggish, have headaches, and see rashes, all of which may be signs of internal damage. While plants and animals are easy enough to avoid, toxic chemicals, substances, poisons, and other hazardous materials may be leaching from your household products. But how do these differ from toxins?

Toxic Chemicals and Substances

A toxic chemical or substance is something that is poisonous to the body but is not necessarily living or comes from plant or animal materials — this would include radon, lead, mercury, and gas. Like many biotoxins, toxic chemicals and substances can produce immediate adverse reactions or long-term damage (such as cancer, liver failure, reproductive issues, etc.). Many household cleaners, products, drugs, cosmetics, and pesticides use these toxic chemicals and substances. Over time, many of these substances leak fumes or come into contact with your skin and are absorbed into your body.

A common toxic substance that you see every day is plastic. It can be found in millions of everyday items, from packaging to household tools. A recent study of a group of random individuals showed that seventy-seven percent of people have microplastics in their bloodstream[2], a number which shouldn't come as a surprise since, *on a weekly basis*, we ingest enough plastic to create a credit card![3] The significance of this long-term is not fully known, although it is thought to affect cells, hormones, and organ function while also contributing to diseases such as cancer.

Poisons

While all toxins are poisons, not all poisons are toxins. As mentioned earlier, a toxin is a natural substance produced by a plant or animal that causes a negative effect on your health. The term poison is a broader term that would include toxins, chemicals, and substances that produce ill effects on health, environment, and property.

Hazardous Materials

A material is considered hazardous when it can cause an extreme physical reaction such as fires, explosions, or gas, mainly when they are mixed or comes into contact with another material or chemical. A hazardous material can be biological, chemical, physical, or radiological. Not all toxins and chemicals are hazardous; however, hazardous materials are often referred to as 'dangerous goods.' There are nine hazardous material classifications:

1. Class 1 – Explosives
2. Class 2 – Compressed or flammable gasses
3. Class 3 – Flammable liquids
4. Class 4 – Flammable solids
5. Class 5 – Oxidizing substances and organic peroxides
6. Class 6 – Toxic and infectious substances
7. Class 7 – Radioactive materials
8. Class 8 – Corrosives
9. Class 9 – Miscellaneous dangerous goods

Toxicity and Toxicity Levels

The toxicity of a substance refers to how toxic (i.e., dangerous) a toxin or poisonous material is. Toxicity is measured through various factors, including the dosage, length of exposure, the effects it produces, and route of exposure.

The dosage of a toxin refers to how much of the toxin a person comes into contact with. For example, a milliliter of gas that accidentally touches your skin while you fuel your car may cause a slight irritation on your skin, while being dosed in gallons of fuel due to a malfunction at the pump could cause severe skin damage, burning of the throat and lungs, and a whole host of other internal injuries (this is a rather extreme example that I hope you never experience!). Therefore, while gas is dangerous, the milliliter that accidentally drips onto your skin will have low or minimal toxicity. In contrast, the gallons of spilled gas would have a high toxicity. In short, toxicity refers to the *amount* of the substance.

Length of exposure refers to how long you are exposed to a toxic material. This can range anywhere from a few seconds to years or decades. The World Health Organization states that in 2019 alone, about one million people died from long-term exposure to lead, and many more millions were debilitated by it.[4]

Sometimes, a one-time exposure may have no short-term or long-term side effects. Some substances immediately produce side effects, whereas others build up over time. The length of exposure can produce side effects such as vomiting, rashes, headaches, cancers, and organ failures.

USING TOXINS

Toxins are dangerous. When using toxins, this should always be at the forefront of your thoughts. Through my experience of readily using products with toxins, by reducing them as much as possible, I have noticed significant improvements in my family's health. If you must use a toxin or a chemical product, consider doing the following to limit your exposure:

- ❖ Wear a hazmat mask and appropriate personal protective equipment (PPE)
- ❖ Wear long sleeves and elbow-length rubber gloves
- ❖ Turn on or increase air filtration systems
- ❖ Don't eat or drink
- ❖ Don't work alone
- ❖ Wash clothes and body after exposure

Call poison control if you begin to feel sick, nauseous, feverish, or experience symptoms such as headaches or rashes. If you think you may need immediate medical attention, phone 9-1-1.

COMMON ENVIRONMENTAL TOXINS

Dr. Jodi Flaws of the University of Illinois recently stated, 'More than 300 environmental contaminants or the metabolic by-products of those contaminants have been measured in human urine, blood or other biological samples.' [5] These toxins extend far beyond just 'common environmental toxins,' and it goes to demonstrate how much more we need to be aware of the toxins around us.

There are thousands of toxins, chemicals, and other harmful substances worldwide, and we can't cover them all due to time and space. However, let's take a closer look at the most commonly interacted with toxins you come into contact with when using everyday items found in your home or at work. For simplicity's sake, we'll refer to toxins, poisons, and chemicals interchangeably.

Asbestos

Asbestos is a common carcinogenic (a substance that may cause cancer) silicate mineral found in many older homes and in building supplies. Because it is heat resistant and lowers the rate of corrosion, at one time, many building materials used asbestos to strengthen the product and add longevity to it. Asbestos is the leading cause (70% of cases) of mesothelioma, an otherwise rare type of lung and abdomen cancer. It is also linked to other types of lung cancers and laryngeal and ovarian cancers.

BPA (Bisphenol A)

In recent years, there has been a considerable outcry against BPA, a substance that makes polycarbonate plastics and resins clear. It is also sometimes found on the interior of metal cans. Everything from plastic water bottles to plastic cutlery to canned food to baby bottles use or have used BPA in their composition. While some businesses and products have moved away from BPA, it is still a prevalent substance.

BPA can leach into food and cause long-term conditions or increase the difficulty of certain diseases such as Type 2 diabetes, obesity, behavioral issues, cardiovascular health, and increased blood pressure. It is particularly concerning for teenagers and women as it has the ability to negatively affect hormones as it mimics estrogen (often referred to as an endocrine disruptor).

While a 2002 study was over twenty years old, it was found that 93% of people contained some amount of BPA in their urine.[6] It would be safe to assume that a very high number would still be present today.

BPS (Bisphenol S)

BPS is less well-known than BPA. However, it is once again a harmful chemical used to make polyether sulfone plastics, which is found in hard plastics, synthetic clothing fibers, textiles, sales receipts, and sometimes in the interior of cans. When BPA is taken out of a product, it is often replaced with BPS and is comparable or sometimes worse in toxicity levels to BPA.

BPS can play a role in causing or increasing the symptoms of conditions such as obesity, gestational diabetes, metabolic disorders, damage to DNA, and breast cancer.[7] A recent study has shown that 81% of Americans have traces of BPS in their urine.[8]

Formaldehyde

Formaldehyde is another carcinogenic compound found in many building supplies and resins. Despite the known dangers it presents to humans, it is still widely used today. Formaldehyde has a strong smell, although it is colorless. Exposure to formaldehyde can cause vision and nasal tenderness, headaches, and a burning sensation in the throat and lungs. It is often referred to as methanal or methylene oxide but is not limited to those names. Frequent symptoms of formaldehyde poisoning include damage to the nervous system.

Lead

Lead is a relatively popular heavy metal with a long history of use tracing back to the ancient Babylonian days. Unfortunately, today, it is still used and considered a common household toxin. It is found in paint (pre-1978) and was also used in water pipes since it resists corrosion. As exposure to lead increases and the body absorbs it, adverse side effects begin to present themselves — this is known as lead poisoning. Symptoms of this include feeling sluggish, diarrhea, constipation, weakness, and vomiting. In severe cases, it can be lethal. Children who are exposed to lead can suffer developmentally.

Mercury

Do you recall using a glass thermometer to check your temperature as a child? If so, most likely, the liquid inside was mercury. Mercury is less common today than it was a few decades ago; however, it can still be found in many lightbulbs, older washers and dryers, and while burning coal or oil. Exposure to mercury or when suffering from mercury poisoning may lead to lung and brain damage with symptoms such as difficulty speaking, memory difficulties, and sensory issues. The most common way to ingest mercury is by eating seafood. Fish, such as tuna, king mackerel, pike, and bass, are all known to often contain mercury.

Methylmercury

There are many different types of mercury, and methylmercury is the most toxic of them all. When mercury is dissolved or added to freshwater or saltwater bodies, methylmercury is created. When aquatic animals digest the methylmercury, it is condensed and transmitted to humans when they eat the aquatic animals. Up to 90% of mercury found in humans is from seafood. Similarly, ranges from 75% to 90% of methylmercury is also from consuming seafood. Because of methylmercury's toxicity, women with methylmercury in their bodies can result in stillbirths or cause developmental deformities in babies still in the womb. Regular exposure or severe doses of methylmercury can cause neurological problems and harm many aspects of cellular functioning.

You may be wondering why the emphasis on methylmercury when mercury was just discussed. Is it that much different or worse than mercury? Let's go back to Iraq in 1971 and the poisoned grain incident. Towards the end of that year, grain treated with methylmercury fungicide was imported into Iraq as seed grain (aka seeds that are meant for planting, not consumption). The seed bags were labeled in Spanish and English, and contained a skull and crossbones symbol, and then were distributed to rural areas (where it can be assumed that very few people knew Spanish, English, or the symbol) as seed grain. Unfortunately, the bags were mistaken as food, and thousands of rural Iraqis consumed the grain. There were 6,350 reported cases of methylmercury poisoning, of which officially 409 people died. However, it is thought that both these numbers are at least ten times higher than what was reported. The poisoning resulted in paralysis, loss of motor skills, cerebral palsy, blindness, and many other conditions and symptoms.

Unfortunately, methylmercury poisoning in the masses has been reported in Japan and Australia, and by sharing these instances with you, which largely have been forgotten today, I hope that we can prevent similar incidents in the future by being very careful about what we put in our bodies.

Phthalates

This carcinogenic chemical is found in hundreds of items at your local grocery store, ranging from shampoos and conditioners to body lotions and fragrances. It is also found in medical supplies, cleaning supplies, and laundry detergents. But why? Phthalates are used to soften plastics, thereby making them flexible or easily dissolvable. It is also used to attach chemicals and scents.

Phthalates have been linked to cancers, hormone disruptions, child growth/development, and causing damage to the liver, lungs, kidneys, and the reproductive system.

Polybrominated diphenyl ethers (PDEs)

Commonly referred to as flame retardants, polybrominated diphenyl ethers is a substance often found in manufactured items that, as its name suggests, quells fires. It is typically found in electronics and insulating materials, two groups of products that have a higher-than-average likelihood of catching fire and accelerating quickly. It is thought that PDEs affect the liver, brain, and thyroid. While PDEs can leak into food, it may be most concerning for firefighters and people who live in areas associated with wildfires.

Polychlorinated biphenyls

While polychlorinated biphenyls have been banned in the USA since the 1970s, unfortunately, they still linger in items such as insulations, coolants, and automotive parts. Over time, this makes its way into the food chain, mainly through fish and meats. Polychlorinated biphenyls are carcinogenic and may cause short-term memory loss in children, negatively affect the thyroid, and present neurological deficiencies.

Cadmium

Zinc production results in a by-product known as cadmium, which is in the top ten most dangerous heavy metals. It has only been in use since the twentieth century and was largely used during the First World War as a substitute for tin. It is mainly used today as a component of rechargeable batteries, although it is sometimes used in paints and protective coatings.

Cadmium is polluted into the air, eventually settling in soil and other organic materials, where it can stay for decades. Fruits and vegetables absorb the cadmium while growing, which is then passed onto humans when they eat the crops.

Arsenic

This toxic chemical is readily found in the earth's crust and makes its way into soil and water systems. Crops grown in soil containing arsenic or watered with water that contains arsenic will absorb the arsenic, which is then passed onto humans. However, the most frequent occurrence of arsenic in humans is from water sources. As much as 7% of wells in the USA contain arsenic, along with many more significant water sources such as lakes and rivers. Since arsenic is tasteless and odorless, water and soil must be tested to determine its presence. Low exposure to arsenic can have an immediate effect on hormones. In contrast, long-term exposure can lead to harm in most of the body's organ systems, including cardiovascular, nervous, respiratory, and immune systems, along with causing damage to organs such as the liver, lungs, and prostate. It can also negatively impact a child's development. Tip: If you are worried about arsenic in your drinking water, many affordable water filters have the capacity to remove it.

Perfluoroalkyl and poly-fluoroalkyl substances (PFAs)

There are over 9,000 PFAs used to prevent food from sticking to pans, containers, and other foods to each other. Because they are built to be water and grease-resistant, it is also challenging for the body to break them down. Consequently, PFAs are sometimes known as 'forever chemicals' given how seldom your body can detox it from its systems. In most countries, organizations and labels do not have to list PFAs on their packaging, making it very difficult to remove them from your life without doing extensive research on your own. However, in future chapters, we will discuss PFAs in more depth and what products to avoid since many of them exist. Research is beginning to show that PFAs are carcinogenic (particularly for kidney and testicular cancers), affect hormones and the thyroid, and can cause heart disease, immune deficiencies, and fetal development issues. And this is just the beginning of all the problems PFAs can cause. As Meg Bohne, associate director of campaigns, Consumer Reports says, "We know unequivocally that PFAS chemicals are contaminating communities and waterways, and putting our health at risk."[9]

Parabens

Popular in beauty and cleaning products, such as soaps, shampoos, cosmetics, and deodorants, parabens are a preservative that has strongly been linked to cancers, particularly breast cancer. Since parabens are primarily used on 'external' body care products, most food and drug agencies do not regulate parabens. Many people have falsely believed that if they don't literally eat something with parabens (or any toxin for that matter), then they won't need to worry about the side effects it causes. However, this is far from the truth. The skin is the body's largest organ, absorbing many toxins, including parabens. For example, when you stand in the shower and wash your hair, your scalp absorbs the parabens, and as you rinse out the soap, it runs over your skin, causing further opportunities for absorption. Deodorants are designed to absorb, and so do many perfumes, lotions, and cosmetics.

Perfluorinated chemicals (PFCs)

PFCs are very similar to PFAs in that they are designed to make items water, grease, and stain-resistant. They are often used in kitchen items, carpets, bedding, and in many industrial enterprises such as automotive, building, electronics, and aerospace. Once PFCs enter your body, it can take years for them to leave the blood. The health consequences of having PFCs in your bloodstream are nearly identical to that of PFAs.

Volatile organic compounds (VOC)

In the world of toxins, the term 'organic' refers to compounds that contain the element carbon. Many toxins are VOCs, which means that when the chemical comes into contact with air or sunlight, it produces toxic waste, greenhouse gasses, or contamination. This has short and long-term health consequences, including irritation to the senses, headaches, allergic reactions, lung damage, kidney failure/damage, etc.

HOUSEHOLD TOXINS?

Are toxins really a concern in products around my house? Unfortunately, they are a bigger problem than you realize. Toxic chemicals are found in thousands of household items ranging from cleaners to body care, to clothes and carpets. In some cases, the toxins are saturated in the materials your home was made with. With the amount of toxins present today, it's no surprise that many people feel tired and sluggish, suffer from skin rashes and acne, have headaches, and overall, just don't feel well. Many chemicals are also associated with unexplainable weight gain and cancers. Toxins could be the root cause or be heavily contributing to the symptoms of your illnesses.

While many toxins are silent and odorless, they can be deadly. Toxins can build up over years, and you will only feel worse without the effort to remove them from your body. It can be tricky to know what is toxic and what's just unpleasant, but I hope to walk you through this in the following chapters after we take a more in-depth look at toxins and your health.

Five Things You Can Do Today:

- ❖ Read labels! With frequent glances at labels, you'll begin to understand what goes into products. This includes items at 'health' food stores or anything listed as 'natural' or 'organic.'
- ❖ Get your water tested for toxins.
- ❖ Survey your home. Make a list of items that may possibly contain toxins. Keep this for future chapters and compare them when you get there.
- ❖ Write down how you feel physically and begin this as a monthly habit to track your health progress as you remove toxins from your life.
- ❖ Research unique items you have in your home to see if they may be contaminated with toxins. This book will cover everyday, common household items, so do some research to ensure that you don't have rare contaminants in your home.

UNDERSTANDING TOXINS & TOXICITY

As we move forward to the next chapter, recall that a toxin is a substance that causes short-term or long-term health problems. These can range from having low toxicity to being deadly in minutes of exposure. Everyday household items are all 'low' in toxicity; however, the slow build-up over time has devastating effects on health as your body struggles to process them. In the next chapter, we will take a further look at why the human body can't handle toxins, how it processes them, and why they are harmful.

2

PROCESSING TOXINS

Zara stared at the scale in disbelief. A week had gone by since the last time she weighed herself. A week of low-calorie diets, exercise, and supplements, only to be rewarded with another pound added to her waistline. Frustrated, she felt a tear come to her eye. She was doing everything, but it seemed to no avail. Why couldn't she lose weight? She had tried everything: keto, Whole30, gluten-free, sugar-free, weight training, supplements, diet pills, protein, and plant-based, intermittent fasting... The list could go on; she would lose five pounds over the last ten years only to gain seven back. In fact, it seemed like her health only got worse as she frequently had gut pain and severe bloating.

Another week went by, and Zara had gained another pound. She was sitting at a local café with a new coworker, Marya, eating a large bowl of greens drizzled in olive oil. Marya took a sip of kombucha and made a face.

"Why are you drinking that if you don't like it?" asked Zara, who rather liked kombucha, confused as to why someone would pay five dollars for something they didn't enjoy.

"It's another source of probiotics," replied Marya. "I've had a lot of health problems over the years, and the probiotics in kombucha and other fermented foods and drinks have been crucial to my recovery."

"Hmmm...," was Zara's only response.

"However," continued Marya, "It was getting rid of toxins that really pushed my health from okay to great. It helped me lose weight, improved my mental health, and my kids, wow, do I ever see a difference in their behaviors, attitudes, and mental abilities!"

Marya now had Zara's full attention, and over the remaining forty minutes of their lunch hour, Zara grilled Marya about how she improved her gut health and removed toxins from her home. Marya patiently answered every query.

In one lunch hour, Zara's life changed more than she ever dreamed could happen. Marya discussed how she didn't want toxins from the old paint and vinyl flooring affecting her children, so she renovated her home to reflect the natural living principles she had adopted, including the removal of obesogens.

Over the next eighteen months, Zara began to make changes to her health by adopting a gut-friendly diet that cured her leaky gut and helped her lose weight, but she also adopted an obesogens-free home. Like Marya, she switched her chemical cleaners for non-toxic ones, and threw out all her scented candles, air fresheners, and antibacterial mouthwash, swapping them all for healthier alternatives.

As Zara learned, toxins were destructive to her health and attempts to lose weight. The toxins were killing the good bacteria in her gut, while her fluctuating diets never focused on balancing her gut bacteria and fixing her gut lining—a condition also known as leaky gut.

In this chapter, we will look at how toxins found in households and the environment affect your gut microbiome and, by extension, your overall health.

An obesogen is a toxic chemical affecting the body's metabolic health by lowering energy outputs, leading to fat cells and fat storage increases, thereby causing weight gain. To date, there have been over fifty toxins identified as obesogens, with the number expected to rise in the coming months and years. Obesogen toxins are concerning as many of them are linked to 'forever chemicals' such as PFA, a common ingredient in many household plastics.

From the moment a child is conceived, they are exposed to obesogens. While food has played a significant role in America's weight gain over the last few decades, obesogens have the ability to affect genes, creating the potential difficulty for generations to come with weight and additional health conditions later in life. One way obesogens play a role in weight gain is that they change the gut microbiota.

Many toxins have the ability to alter hormones (i.e., chemical messengers), and these endocrine disruptors affect everything from reproductive health to digestion and to your mood.

HOW TOXINS IMPACT US

Like Marya, Zara lived in an older home. Over the years, Zara and her husband had done a few renovations, but overall, Zara loved the character and made only a few minimal changes to her home. Once she discovered how toxic paint could be, Zara immediately sent in paint chips to check for toxins — and they came back *very* positive.

No one thinks that paint will make you sick, but when it is decades old and from a time when toxins weren't known (or considered), then unknowingly, you could be living in the presence of toxins that disrupt your endocrine system. Hundreds of toxic chemicals affect this system, which includes the pituitary gland, thyroid gland, parathyroid gland, adrenal gland, pancreas, ovaries, testes, adipose tissue (also known as fat tissue), kidneys, and gut.

Endocrine-disrupting compounds (EDC) are amalgams that interfere with, block, or mimic hormones.[1] This is very concerning for women as it affects menstrual cycles, reproduction capabilities, pregnancies, and menopause. In short, a toxin with endocrine-disrupting capabilities plays a massive role in our lives when we allow toxins to be part of it. As one report stated so succinctly, 'Hormones are critical to reproduction. ... EDCs block connections between these hormones and their receptors, or they mimic hormonal activity, thereby tricking a hormone receptor into action. Either way, EDCs interfere with the normal function of hormonal systems.' [2] The same report stated the sad reality of EDCs, 'Exposure to EDCs has been linked to structural and functional impairments of reproductive systems.' [3] Thousands of women suffer from infertility and endometritis—and without a doubt, reducing toxic chemi-

PROCESSING TOXINS

cals with endocrine-disrupting compounds would be a significant first step to improving their reproductive (and overall!) health.

One of the most commonly used endocrine system toxins is PFA— perfluoroalkyl and poly-fluoroalkyl substances—of which there are over 9,000 and can be found in tens of thousands of household items. Other products in the home that disrupt the endocrine system include alkylphenols, atrazine, phthalates, organotins, and halogenated flame retardants.

But many more toxins affect the endocrine system, and 'household exposure studies ... show that people are exposed to complex mixtures of indoor toxins from building materials and a myriad of consumer products.' [4] The variety of toxins in homes is just beginning to be understood, and their impacts on future generations are not yet known. Taking care of your body not only affects you, but it will change your family tree.

There is something that is referred to as the 'one percent rule.' The basic concept of it is if you improve yourself by one percent every day, then, while progress won't be noticed on a day-to-day basis, within a year, you'll have improved by 37.78 percent. Why is it effective? Because a slight improvement every day is doable and brings lasting changes. The same is true for the opposite. If you feel one percent worse every day, you won't notice it immediately, but you will over months and years. Low toxicity exposure is similar. The gradual increase in toxins doesn't hit you like a brick; instead, you slowly feel it over time, often unaware that the toxins surrounding you make you feel this way. You chalk it up to stress, work, lack of exercise, or getting older. Across all the known toxins, they affect every bodily function from the cellular level to organs and blood.

Every bodily function can be affected by toxins. That is why they are so damaging to your health.

Removing toxins from the home is like purifying your hormonal system. Day by day, as you remove toxins from your home, say one percent at a time, your hormonal system will respond positively in time. It's time to start changing your life.

THE GUT

The gut microbiome is your 'second brain' as it affects digestion, physical health, mental health, and all systems of the body. When the gut microbiome is healthy, it positively affects these areas of health; when it is not, there is a good chance that these areas will suffer.

The gut microbiome is made up of about one hundred trillion microorganisms, such as bacteria, fungi, and viruses, which can loosely be divided into good and bad microorganisms. The bulk of these are found in the large intestine. Even the best microbiome in the world contains both types; however, a healthy gut must have far more healthy microorganisms than bad ones. A healthy gut also doesn't have any holes in the intestinal lining, also known as a 'leaky gut.'

A healthy, diverse microbiome plays a crucial role in heart, weight, immune system health, and hormone regulation. They are responsible for breaking down different vitamins and minerals and then converting that into energy for the rest of your body to use; this ranges from improving cellular activity to producing neurotransmitters that improve your mood.

The microbiome begins to develop during birth as a baby passes through the birth canal. From there, its diversity grows through breast milk, and then as the baby grows into a child and into its teenage years, it continues to grow and expand in diversity, mainly through food but also through the environment. The immune system and the microbiome are then intrinsically connected, and about 70% of the immune system is found in the gut. An unhealthy diet filled with processed foods, lack of exercise, poor sleep, and antibiotics will all destroy the healthy microorganisms, ultimately leading to various health problems and weight gain.

A diverse, healthy microbiome can be built over time through good lifestyle habits and food. Lifestyle habits include getting enough sleep, exercising four to five times a week, and reducing stress. Probiotic foods contain microorganisms that contribute to the gut microbiome, such as yogurt, sauerkraut, kombucha, and kimchi — in short, fermented foods. In order for the probiotic foods to thrive, they need to be fed 'prebiotics. Prebiotic foods are certain fruits and vegetables, typically high in fiber, that cultivate the growth of good bacteria in our gut. The next step would be to avoid foods with toxins, namely prepackaged foods, and fruits and vegetables sprayed with chemicals.

TOXINS AND THE GUT

Without a doubt, toxins destroy healthy gut microorganisms. There are two main groups these toxins can be found in: food and environment. When toxins are digested, they kill good bacteria (while also damaging the liver, kidneys, and other critical organs), allowing the bad bacteria to grow and take over your gut intestines. While it is very easy to kill good bacteria, it is much more challenging to build it back up again. As one report states, 'Certain environmental toxins can induce damage and dysfunction in the liver, which is termed as liver toxicity. Exposure to these toxins changes the liver's morphology and functionality, leading to liver diseases. Similarly, exposure to some environmental chemicals causes structural differences and functional alterations in the gut microbiome ... For instance, arsenic exposure can perturb the composition and metabolites of the mouse gut microbiome, which potentially contributes to its toxicity.' [5]

TOXINS THAT AFFECT THE GUT

As mentioned earlier, there are thousands of toxic chemicals, many of which directly impact your gut microbiome. The following list touches on some common toxins people frequently use or have in their homes. These all damage the gut microbiome, and their additional health costs have also been noted. Tip: Bookmark this page for future reference so that you have a quick cheat sheet of things to remove from your home!

1. Bleach. From cleaning supplies to laundry detergent, bleach is a cheap toxin that many people have in their homes. When you pop open the lid of a bleach bottle, you are instantly hit with toxic fumes known to cause asthma and pneumonia. It increases your risk for COPD (chronic obstructive pulmonary disease) by 25% and can cause damage to the liver, which is responsible for breaking down and digesting fats.

2. Antibacterial Chemicals. Covid-19 taught us to use hand sanitizer all the time to avoid germs. However, it can also kill the good bacteria on our skin, weakening our systems as the bad bacteria thrive. The same goes for most household cleaners and toothpaste.

3. Dry-Cleaning Chemicals. The chemicals used to clean the clothes are much worse than the laundry detergents found on the grocery shelf as they cause damage to the kidney, liver, and nervous system.

4. Vinyl Floorings. Vinyl flooring, especially rolls, had become very popular due to its water-resistant properties and affordability. However, it has been linked to liver, brain, breast, and lung cancer. While most of us can't just replace our flooring, we can move towards safer practices such as not sitting or lying on vinyl floors and laying child-safe mats down in playrooms. When the time comes to change your floor, look for better options.

5. Triclosan. There are some ingredients that you just want to shout from the rooftops not to touch — and triclosan is one of those. Triclosan is concerning because it damages the immune-building activities microbes undertake. In order to be healthy and stay healthy for years to come, your immune system needs to be strong, and triclosan will only fight against your immune system's health.

6. Flame Retardants. Another dangerous chemical often found in mattresses, baby car seats, and foam cushions, flame retardants can damage the endocrine system, cause cancer, and hinder child development.

7. Pesticides. Pesticides might kill the pesky weed but are found in high doses in non-organic meats. It kills weeds but also good bacteria. More on these can be found in chapter three.

8. Non-Stick Chemicals. Also known as PFOAs or PFAs, non-stick chemicals can cause significant reproduction damage. See Chapter One for more information.

9. Baby Powder. Perhaps not a household item you thought to see on this list, but baby powder is highly toxic to both babies and women. It has been directly linked to lung damage. The severity of this chemical is such that hundreds of millions of dollars are awarded yearly to those who used it in the past and suffered long-term consequences from it.

10. BPA. This chemical poses a severe risk to the hormonal system. See Chapter One for more information about BPA.

The list above is relatively short and in no way can fully represent the extensive damage of the thousands of toxins that could be found in the home that could ruin your gut microbiota. But beyond toxins, antibiotics, heavy metals, preservatives, pesticides, and genetically modified foods can all play a role in gut health.

Toxins destroy your gut health, which, in turn, has a devastating effect. Suzy Kassem highlighted the dangers of it best when she said, 'Polluting the gut not only cripples your immune system but also destroys your sense of empathy, the ability to identify with other humans. Bad bacteria in the gut create neurological issues. Autism can be cured by detoxifying the bellies of young children. People who think that feelings come from the heart are wrong. The gut is where you feel the loss of a loved one first. It's where you feel pain and a heavy bulk of your emotions. It's the central base of your entire immune system. If your gut is loaded with negative bacteria, it affects your mind...' [6] While we do not know everything about autism nor whether detoxing and nutrition are the complete answer to resolving the illness, what we do know for a fact is that it is always better for your overall health.

CHILDREN & TOXINS

Red food dye 40: made from petroleum and approved by the U.S. Food and Drug Administration as safe for human consumption. It is used in many processed and prepackaged foods, including cereals, candy, sodas, pastries, yogurts, snacks, and desserts. In other words, the aisle at the grocery store where you shop for your children's snacks—bright, colorful snacks to appeal to children—is filled with red food dye (and many other dyes!). While the color may be appealing, the side effects are not: ADHD, allergies, behavioral problems, depression, sensory irritations, and headaches.

Red food dye is just one of the many toxins found in food.[7] Millions of children today are diagnosed with ADD and ADHD, and when we look at the side effects just one dye or toxin has, it should come as no surprise. However, thousands of people have also reported that they removed this dye from their children's diet and switched out household cleaners and self-care products. They have seen considerable improvements in their children's behavior in just one to two weeks.

The toxin commonly referred to as BPA is also particularly harmful to children as BPA can leak into food. This can have a detrimental effect on the brain and prostate gland of children ranging from unborn babies to early teenage years. It has also been linked to behavioral issues. [8] Another toxin, phthalates, has been linked to miscarriages, developmental delays, obesity, allergies, and reproductive hormonal damage.

Why do toxins have such an amplified impact on children? Children are vulnerable to toxins primarily due to their small size. They often absorb similar amounts of toxins compared to adults; however, the bodies are usually just a small percentage of an adult's body. Children often touch toys and put various objects and their hands in their mouths, making it very easy for them to ingest toxins. Over the last two decades, childhood cancers have risen by twenty percent, and the only explanation seems to be the continual rise in toxins.

In the Western world, we expect drinking water to be safe. Communities in cities like Flint, Michigan, are known to have lead-contaminated water, and yet parents can't afford to move, and city councils seem uninterested in fixing the problem. The problems continue today.

Children thrive in the environment that you create for them. They don't understand words like 'toxins' and 'cancer' or what is safe to put in their mouth. Detoxing your home is more than just for your health; it sets your children's health up for success.

With a clear understanding of what toxins are and how they damage your health, let's dive into practical ways you can detox your home. In Part Two, we will cover all the general areas of your home and the different toxins and toxic household products you may have in those areas. Let's begin eliminating and minimizing toxins in your home!

Five Things You Can Do Today

❖ Incorporate more gut-healthy, probiotic food into your diet and avoid foods with toxins. This means adding fermented foods, grass-fed/organically raised meat (opposed to those from the factory-farmed system) and eating organic whole foods.
❖ Throw out all plastics marked with a '7' — numbers two, four, and five are the safest plastics.

❖ Wash your hands with soap more often. Especially after touching potential toxins and being in unsanitary conditions.
❖ Say goodbye to red dye 40. No exceptions.
❖ Add more fruits and vegetables to your diet.

PART II

THE ACTION PLAN

3

DETOX: THE KITCHEN AND DINING ROOM

> *"Regular exposure to the galaxy of chemicals we encounter daily poses a potential health hazard. About 90,000 human-made chemicals now exist, and we don't know how daily exposure to them affects our health. Some precaution is reasonable, and the kitchen is a good place to start..."* [1]
>
> — TOM PERKINS, THE GUARDIAN

Chemicals. Toxins. Poisons. Contaminants. Pollutants. These are the modern-day killers of health. Despite living in an age where we have access to more information and healthy goods than ever before, the number of people with cancer, heart disease, obesity, and poor gut health continues on an upward trajectory. However, this does not need to be part of your story: It's time to change your future, and that begins in the heart of the home — the kitchen.

The kitchen is my domain and happy place. It's where I make nutritious meals for my family, where my kids bake cookies for me, and create so many happy memories. Despite how long a day may feel, I know that at the end of it, I am surrounded by my family in the dining room, enjoying our last meal of the day together. It's filled with odd squabbles and occasionally a few tears, but most days, it's a place where we bond, laughing and talking about our crazy days.

While my family often doesn't consider the atmosphere, it brings me great peace and joy to know that we have eliminated many of the toxins commonly found in the kitchen and dining room.

TOXINS PRESENT

A hundred years ago, a kitchen had one or two pots, a few ladles, cups, plates, and cutlery. Today, it's only when you move homes you realize how many kitchen items you have accumulated over the years. From cutlery to kitchen gadgets, the average kitchen has over one thousand items packed into just a few hundred square feet.

Big bulk stores like Walmart and Target have made it easy and convenient to pick up an item or two while shopping. Then along came dollar and discount stores filled with even more ultra-low priced items. Finally, Amazon came along, and with a click of a mouse, we had the world of supplies at our fingertips without ever having to step past the front door.

Is it our fault that our kitchens (and, by default, our homes) have so much stuff? I argue that it's not. Our willpower is against billion-dollar corporations with endless marketing funds and research. It takes a very strong person to resist time and time and again.

Despite the ease of access we have to products, the one thing most of us didn't sign up for is getting sick because of the things we have. Let's take a closer look at the toxins and toxic items frequently found in kitchens.

PFAs and PFCs*[2]

Two of my least favorite toxins in the kitchen are perfluoroalkyl and polyfluoroalkyl substances and perfluorinated chemicals, also known as 'forever chemicals,' which are found in thousands of variants. They have been linked to damage in many parts of the reproductive system, high blood pressure, fetal development, thyroid disease, and kidney cancer.

Found In:	Alternative/Solution:
Nonstick pans	Stainless steel, ceramic, and cast iron pans
Nonstick cookware (sheet pans, loaf pans, etc.)	Ceramic, glass, or silicone, stainless steel pans
Plastic cooking utensils	Wooden (hardwood beech, teak, or maple), stainless steel or silicone
Food packaging (candy wrappers, plastic bags, pizza boxes, microwave popcorn)	Shop at zero-waste stores, avoid individually wrapped items, or reduce Make air-popped popcorn at home
Tap water	Water filter: bottle or fridge
Fast food containers	Bring your own glass containers or transfer immediately to glass containers when you get home
Plastic containers	Glass, stainless steel, or silicone
Stain resistant carpets	Natural fiber floor coverings
Plastic cutlery and disposable dishes	Stainless steel, or wooden, and PFA free disposable dishes

While nonstick pans can be convenient, they are not worth the cost of poor health. Instead, using a stainless-steel pan, heat the pan over medium heat for three to five minutes and use a good amount of ghee, butter, or coconut oil to avoid the food from sticking. A frequently asked question is: How safe is ceramic and enamel? Ceramics are safe when they are made of 100% ceramic; anything less may contain lead, another toxin. They can handle heat up to 500F. You can also use ceramic and enamel-coated pots and pans if the coating has not been removed or chipped. Only buy from reputable companies to avoid lead contamination.

An Interim Solution

As we go through the many items found in our homes that contain toxins, you'll begin to understand that it may take some time to replace toxic items with safer items. Therefore, where possible, if I have any solutions you can implement until you can afford replacement items, I will include them in this section labeled as 'An Interim Solution.'

- Sheet pans — cover the bottom with unbleached parchment paper.
- Muffin tins — there are very few options for safe alternatives. Therefore, consider making loaves or using paper (non-bleached) baking cups. Another option is silicone, which thus far research has indicated to be safe and doesn't leach into food so long as it isn't exposed to temperatures above 425 F—which would be a rather high temperature to bake muffins!
- Stain-resistant carpets - place air purifiers nearby to remove any off-gassing from the carpets, open windows more often, and bring in air-purifying plants.

Bisphenol (BPA)*

Linked to hormonal imbalances, neurological conditions, cardiovascular problems, cancer, and Type 2 diabetes, BPA is a prevalent ingredient in the makeup of many kitchen supplies. It is often found abundantly in plastic containers, plastic cutting boards, plastic utensils, plastic cookware, and canned foods.

Found In:	Alternative/Solution:
Plastic cooking utensils	Wooden (hardwood beech, teak, or maple), stainless steel or silicone
Food packaging (plastic bags and containers)	Shop at zero-waste stores and avoid individually wrapped items, reduce consumption of junk foods
Tap water	Water filter: pitcher or fridge
Plastic containers	Glass, stainless steel, ceramic containers
Plastic cutlery and disposable dishes	Stainless steel, camping supplies, travel case with stainless steel utensils
Cutting boards	Bamboo, hardwood, stone, or glass.
Canned food, canned drinks	Food preserved in glass jars, tomato sauce in glass, BPA-free cans Fresh, dried, or frozen fruits and vegetables
Plastic water bottles	Glass with silicone sleeve, stainless steel
Baby bottles	Glass with silicone sleeve, stainless steel, silicone bottle nipples
Plastic coffee makers	Glass French press
Receipts	Opt for digital receipts, or take pictures of receipts then discard, and always wash hands after handling receipts and before eating

While non-BPA products are becoming more available, they are still prevalent, especially among lower-quality items. Plastics with the recycle symbol with a three or seven in them often contain BPA. Also, remember that while a product may be listed as BPA-free, it may contain other—sometimes even worse toxins—in them.

Another thing to take note of is to avoid painted kitchen tools, whether they be glasses or ceramics, as these could contain a variety of toxins.

An Interim Solution

The risk of BPA leaching into your food magnifies when you heat plastic containers, such as in the microwave or in a dishwasher. Over time, heat breaks down plastics, weakening them while increasing the risk of toxin transfer. Always handwash plastic items. As with many other toxins found in plastics, avoid reheating food in plastic containers as it can cause them to seep into the food. Instead, place food in glass bowls or ceramic bowls.

Phthalates*

This toxin has largely been known to be an endocrine disruptor and is linked to asthma, ADHD, male fertility issues, cancer, and obesity. It is commonly found in dish soaps, all-purpose cleaners, and detergents, along with their alternatives (many brands are beginning to carry non-toxic cleaners!). It is also commonly found in plastic wraps, PVC plumbing pipes, and plastic kitchen supplies.

Found In:	Alternative/Solution:
Plastic cooking utensils	Wooden (hardwood beech, teak, or maple), silicone or steel
Plastic plumbing pipes	When it is time to change plumbing infrastructure (such as during renovations or new builds), look into safer options such as copper or galvanized steel pipes.
Plastic containers	Glass, stainless steel, silicone or porcelain containers
Plastic cutlery and throwaway dishes	Stainless steel, camping supplies
Cutting boards	Bamboo, hardwood, stone, or glass
Vinyl flooring	Wood, natural fiber carpets

Some foods are exceptionally high in phthalates because of their packaging; this includes restaurant and fast food eateries, infant formulas, processed foods, cooking oils, and high-fat animal products.

Bleach

Bleach is corrosive, a combination of water and sodium hypochlorite. It is a powerful cleaner and disinfectant, killing viruses, bacteria, and germs — but also good microorganisms needed for gut health. Exposure to bleach can cause skin rashes, a burning sensation in the throat and lungs, and chlorine poisoning.

Found In:	Alternative/Solution:
Household bleach	Vinegar and lemon essential oil, baking soda, oxygen-based bleach, leaving clothes out in the sun
Household cleaners	Warm water, vinegar, essential oils, oxygen-based bleach

Lead*

Lead poisoning is unfortunately more common than one would expect due to lead being found in tap water. This can cause neurological conditions—such as cognitive, low IQ levels, behavioral issues, increased blood pressure, anemia, and reproductive issues.

Found In:	Alternative/Solution:
Ceramic mugs and bakeware (that is not 100% ceramic)	Glass, 100% ceramic, stainless steel. Purchase lead testing kits
Older crockpots and slow cookers	Newer items, search for lead-free slow cookers
Paint	Lead-free paint
Water	Water filters: pitcher to fridge

Paint is found not only on walls but also as decoration on bowls, plates, and cups. If you suspect that lead paint may be on the walls in your kitchen (an area that is often warm and damp, causing paint to chip or peel), do not try to scrape it off but rather cover it with a blocker and then a fresh coat of paint — lead-free of course. However, contact a professional construction consultant for the absolute safest removal methods for advice and help.

Aluminum

How many times have you cooked or grilled food on aluminum foil only to have it stick to the food when it's done? As much as you try to peel it off, there is always a remnant of it on the food. Unfortunately, aluminum is strongly linked to dementia and kidney diseases.

Found In:	Alternative/Solution:
Aluminum pots	Stainless steel, ceramic, or cast iron
Aluminum foil	Bleach-free parchment paper, cooking oils and fats, wax paper for wrapping food
Aluminum bottles	Glass or stainless steel

Aluminum produces an added risk as it reacts with acidic foods such as tomatoes and vinegar, causing the aluminum ions to leach into the food at much higher rates.

Preservatives & Additives

For centuries, humans have been preserving food for future months when fresh vegetables, fruits, and meat are scarce. Preservation methods prevent food from spoiling because of various bacteria, oxygen, enzymes, and other microorganisms that could cause the food to decay rapidly. Up until about a hundred years ago, this was done by canning, pickling, and

DETOX: THE KITCHEN AND DINING ROOM

drying, using a variety of salts, spices, and vinegar. Ingredients such as alcohol and citric acid were also occasionally used. Today, millions of households still use these methods to prepare food for long-term use, but many more don't.

The traditional methods of preserving food have long been substituted for artificial preservatives that benefit large corporations' pocketbooks at the expense of health. Artificial preservatives can increase the shelf life of a product by months or years, thereby allowing businesses to be less concerned about immediate product turnover and consumption; whether the product stays on the shelf for two days or four days is rather indifferent to them so long as the product is purchased within a reasonable amount of time and doesn't result in so-called 'food' waste.

Another critical reason for preservatives is that it helps to preserve the look and texture of the food. Preservatives are used in food found in grocery stores and fast food restaurants.

One artificial preservative commonly used to preserve meat is nitrate, a preservative that is linked to colon cancer. MSG, short for monosodium glutamate, is a popular additive many people know about and desire to avoid. High fructose corn syrup is found in many processed sugar snacks and is another villain we best avoid, as it's been known to lead to diabetes and obesity. Two other culprits are butylated hydroxyanisole (BHA) and butylated hydroxytoluene (BHT), which cause neurological deficiencies and are carcinogenic — these are often added to chips, highly processed vegetable oils, gum, and breakfast cereals.

Found In:	Alternative/Solution:
Frozen boxed meals	Fresh made-from-scratch meals
Instant foods	Dried foods and snacks, fresh fruits and vegetables
	Choose foods with minimal ingredients, and that you can understand
Canned foods	Read all labels very carefully, and ensure BPA-free cans.

We live in a very busy world, and for many people, the accessibility of fast food and easy convenience foods have a certain attraction to them. Like many people, I enjoy a nice meal at a restaurant or going through a drive-through, on occasion, for a quick snack while on the go; sometimes the convenience is needed! However, what I try not to do is to make it a habit or a requirement of my daily life. While I by no means criticize people for wanting an easy option, there is one particular service that has become popular that makes eating fresh easier: meal service plans. There are several options available to choose from, including organic, non-GMO fruits, vegetables, and meals. They come with simple recipes, and groceries, and arrive on your doorstep weekly. While I'm not a fan of all of the packaging, it is a good option if you cannot meal plan, and shop on your own.

Pesticides & Herbicides

Like preservatives, pesticides and herbicides are to be avoided at all costs. These toxins have been designed to kill insects and microorganisms that may touch the food. The question should be, if a pesticide or herbicide has the ability to kill a bug, won't it have the ability to kill cells and negatively impact organs and systems? Indeed, they can.

With more than seventeen thousand pesticides and herbicides, their extensive damage to our bodies is in the infant stages of understanding. But what we do know is that in the short term, they can cause skin irritations, coughing, headaches, and many other flu-like symptoms. In the long term, just to name a few, they can cause cancer, depression, coma, neurological damage, infertility, and organ failure.

The Dirty Dozen

There are some fruits and vegetables that are notorious for the amount of chemicals they contain. In the natural health world, these have been given the nickname of 'The Dirty Dozen.' In short, they highlight twelve of the most polluted crops. While the list changes annually (along with that of the 'Clean Fifteen'), most of the produce on this list remains on it — visit the Environmental Working Group's website, ewg.org, for the latest data.

A frequent misconception is that washing produce removes toxins. Unfortunately, it has been shown time and again that over 75% of washed products still contain toxic chemicals.

1. Apples
2. Bell peppers
3. Blueberries
4. Cherries
5. Grapes
6. Green beans
7. Leafy greens
8. Nectarines
9. Peaches
10. Pears
11. Spinach
12. Strawberry

The Clean Fifteen

In contrast to polluted crops, the clean fifteen refers to the safest fruits and vegetables to consume if you cannot afford to purchase them organically. As you study the list, you will notice that most of these crops have a thick outer layer that is not consumed or are root crops. Overall, these crops have heartier produce and are more resistant to damage, thereby requiring fewer pesticides. Fruits and vegetables that require peeling take many of the toxic chemicals with them when the peels are discarded, and root crops have some protection from the soil against chemicals being directly sprayed onto the food portion of the plant.

1. Asparagus
2. Avocados
3. Cabbage
4. Carrots
5. Honeydew melon
6. Kiwi
7. Mangos
8. Mushrooms
9. Onions
10. Papaya
11. Pineapple
12. Sweetcorn
13. Sweet peas
14. Sweet potatoes
15. Watermelon

Genetically Modified Organisms (GMOs)

GMOs were introduced to create higher-yielding crops that are more efficient by being drought, weed, and pest-resistant while being pesticide and herbicide-friendly. In grocery stores, GMO produce labels begin with the number eight when they are genetically modified; however, applying this label is optional, making it difficult to know when products are not labeled if they are genetically modified.

Many large commercial crops use GMO seeds — this would include corn, soybean, canola, alfalfa, sugar beets, some apples, and other items, but can also be found in everything, from infant formulas, and condiments to supplements. GMO crops are heavily sprayed with herbicides and pesticides. They were designed to resist glyphosate.

Glyphosate, a popular herbicide used with GMO seeds, is so frequently used that it is now found in trace amounts of non-GMO products such as organic and non-GMO produce through cross-contamination. Pests face the immediate consequence of GMO products as when they eat a GMO, it causes holes in the lining of their stomachs, slowly killing them. The human body is thousands of times larger than pests, and our stomachs are stronger than pests (thankfully so!), but damage is being done to our body — leaky gut has become a common diagnosis today, and yet "the experts" claim they don't know the cause of it. Another consequence is the rise in food allergies. Is it right to allow corporations to do this to us? No, it is not. Nutrient deficiencies are subtle, but they cause the body to be off balance, causing hosts of issues ranging from cardiovascular disease to cancer to malnutrition.

Found In:	Alternative/Solution:
Fruits, vegetables, meat, processed foods	Non-GMO crops. Look for a non-GMO certification on labels.[3] Shop at local farmer's markets and develop relationships with the vendors to understand their agriculture practices. Buy organic produce or refer to the Clean 15, and buy organic meat

In her book, Organic Manifesto: How Organic Farming Can Heal Our Planet, Feed the World, and Keep Us Safe, Maria Rodale writes, "Organic is something we can all partake of and benefit from. When we demand organic, we are demanding poison-free food. We are demanding clean air. We are demanding pure, fresh water. We are demanding soil that is free to do its job and seeds that are free of toxins ... buy organic whenever we can, insist on organic, fight for organic and work to make it the norm." This is the approach we need when it comes to toxins in our food and in household products. We must act today to preserve our health and that of our children.

We can change the future if we start today.

Proper Food Storage & Cleaning

Before we move to the next chapter, let's spend a moment discussing one toxin connected to your kitchen: bacteria. Bacteria is typically not a toxin in itself but produces toxins. Like mold, it can be hazardous to our health. The kitchen contains many types of living organisms, often brought in through food. When food waste (think of those Tupperware containers sitting at the back of the fridge for weeks, if not months) is not discarded properly or cleaned up adequately, it can develop bacteria. Add to that the heat and moisture cooking and cleaning brings, and it becomes a breeding ground for bacteria — and not the good kind.

DETOX: THE KITCHEN AND DINING ROOM

On top of that, eating food that has started to go bad or has developed some harmful bacteria can lead to food poisoning. Getting over a bout of food poisoning can be challenging, and while most cases will be resolved within 48 hours, others may take much longer. So, when in doubt, throw out the food that may have gone off.

A few useful tools in the kitchen are to be noted: sponges, tea towels, and cleaning clothes. These items are constantly in contact with food and wet surfaces. After a mess, we clean counters with cleaning clothes and use them to scrub off dirt and wipe down surfaces. We use sponges to wipe food particles and grease off dishes, pots, pans, and everything in between.

We then use tea towels to ensure that everything is dry. However, what do you do with these items when you are done? Many people throw them in the sink or leave them in a wet puddle. However, when they are not dried properly, they become a breeding ground for bacteria. Especially sponges, which never fully get dry and have food particles stuck within their nooks and crannies. These moist, dirty items can become a breeding ground for:

- Staphylococcus aureus: linked to joint pain, abscesses, and pneumonia.
- Enterobacter: linked to UTI, eye and skin infections, and respiratory problems.
- Klebsiella: linked to infections in the lungs, bladder, and brain.
- E. coli: abdominal pain, vomiting, and UTIs.
- Pseudomonas aeruginosa: lung ailments.
- Bacillus subtilis: Eye infections.

At the end of every day, it is essential to clean your kitchen to prevent illnesses and bacteria from growing and spreading. Don't leave old food sitting around or allow wet cloths and sponges to stay damp and breed bacteria. Replace sponges for quick-drying options like dish nets. Have an open area to hang all wet towels, such as a rack or from a hook. Store your kitchen-related cloths in a designated laundry basket or a wet bag, and aim to wash them once a week.

Frequent cleaning of the kitchen and rags will ward off germs, any unwanted stenches, and illnesses related to them.

Toxins can be found everywhere in your kitchen and dining room, from the tools in the drawers to the food you eat. The list may seem endless, but as you transition to a safer kitchen, know that it will have an impact on your health. Use the list above as a starting point and aim to change at least one item every month in your kitchen.

Top Five Things to Do Today:

- ❖ Purchase a water filter and filter all drinking water.
- ❖ Replace all nonstick pans with stainless steel, cast-iron pans, or ceramic.
- ❖ Remove chemical cleaners for plant-based cleaners. You'll find a list at the end of the book.
- ❖ Never put plastics in the microwave or the dishwasher, as this breaks down the chemicals in the plastics, causing them to leach into food.
- ❖ Buy the best quality food you can afford. When possible, aim for organic, non-GMO fruits and vegetables and grass-fed, organic animal products.

4

DETOX: THE BATHROOM & LAUNDRY ROOM

Lead compounds were an essential element of many paints up until 1978. Forty-five years ago, lead-based paint was used almost exclusively for trim work, wainscoting, and high-gloss wall surfaces—such as those found in kitchens and bathrooms. If your home was built before 1978, there is a good chance that it does contain lead-based paint, and it is just one of the many ways toxins have entered the home.

Like the kitchen, in the average home, the bathroom and laundry room are filled with toxins. But rest assured, there are just as many ways to remove, eliminate, or minimize your exposure to them.

TOXINS PRESENT

In pre-toxin awareness days, the mindset is often to 'buy what gets the job done' without a second thought of what harm the product could cause to you. In many ways, we are far too trusting with companies — and perhaps at times, we even rely on the government to restrict products that are unsafe to be in the home or part of your diet. Unfortunately, this is not the case, and we must rely on ourselves to research and determine if something is actually safe or not.

Some of the following toxins found in bathrooms and laundry rooms are a repeat of the previous chapter; however, we will now speak of them in regards to how they relate to items found in these rooms.

Phthalates*[1]

Just as phthalates are found in every room of your home, the illnesses, symptoms, and conditions they cause are vast, ranging from asthma to ADHD, from breast cancer to male fertility issues, and from obesity to neurological disorders. With such potential consequences, we would rather not have them in our homes!

Many scented items, such as soaps and laundry detergents, contain phthalates. Opting for scent-free items will help to reduce the number of phthalates in the cleaning products. Still, the safest measure is always to purchase green, eco-friendly items or to create your own (see the bonus chapter for recipes on my favorite DIY and toxic-free green recipes!).

Found In:	Alternative/Solution:
Laundry detergent	Organic, plant-based detergents
	Natural home cleaners (see bonus chapter for more information!)
Shower curtains	Hemp or 100% cotton shower curtains, glass shower doors
PVC (plastic plumbing pipes)	Copper pipes

DETOX: THE BATHROOM & LAUNDRY ROOM

Shower curtains are both a blessing and a curse. While they keep water from being flung around the bathroom, they can contain toxins in their fabric (whether they are cloth or plastic), but they can also develop toxins such as mold if they are not washed regularly and never dry out. Since bathrooms are naturally damp places, try to regularly open the bathroom window or one nearby that would allow airflow around the curtain to help dry out the area quickly. Along the same line, be sure to turn on the bathroom fan during baths and showers and until after all humidity has left the bathroom. Not only will this help to prevent mold from developing, but it will also prevent paint from peeling and water stains on the walls. If your bathroom doesn't have a built-in fan, bring in a portable fan to get the air moving. A more expensive but arguably the safest option would be to swap out the curtain for glass shower doors. Shower doors can be purchased or custom-made, relatively inexpensive compared to many other home improvement projects — even half doors are available to fit over bathtubs!

Volatile Organic Compound (VOC)*

Despite the term' organic,' volatile organic compounds are not safe. In this instance, organic means a toxin that contains the element carbon. In short, a VOC is a gas resulting from a substance or process. One of the most common VOCs is formaldehyde, but also fuel products such as gas, coal, wood, and kerosene produce VOCs when burned. VOCs have severe consequences, including the sensation of burning (eyes, nose, throat), various kinds of cancer, and damage to the nervous system, liver, and kidneys. In ordinary everyday household items, they are found in cosmetics, hairspray, perfumes, deodorant, glues, toilet bowl cleaners, and some laundry detergents.

In previous decades, smoking was relatively popular, and unfortunately, secondhand smoke contained many pollutants, including VOCs, resulting in lung cancer for many millions of people.

Dryer sheets are another household item that contains VOCs. Dryer sheets are not a necessary part of drying laundry but instead are used as a convenient substitute to reduce static and add a 'clean' smell. But how does it work? Dryer sheets contain a thin layer of wax, which is then slightly warmed/melted by the heat in the dryer; this is then transferred to the clothes to prevent it from sticking. Not only is this wax layer harmful to your body and clothes, but it also builds up over time in the dryer. It can prevent the lint holder from gathering lint (thereby also causing it to get excessively hot in the dryer) and damaging the internal sensors. My personal favorite alternative is wool dryer balls — they are readily available at most home goods stores and online at very affordable prices.

Found In:	Alternative/Solution:
Dryer sheets	Wool dryer balls
Petroleum-based laundry detergents	Unscented, or essential oil scented plant-based detergents and using essential oils to add a scent
Cosmetics	Plant-based and organic cosmetics
Perfumes	Essential oils
Deodorant	Deodorant rocks, all-natural deodorants
Toilet bowl cleaner	Plant-based cleaners, or DIY toilet bowl cleaner (see the bonus section for a recipe!)

Triclosan

Triclosan is a popular ingredient used to make cleaners, soaps, and self-care items antibacterial. It is also found in items not regulated by the Food and Drug Administration, such as children's toys, clothing, furniture, and household items. Slow long-term exposure or a sudden high dose can disrupt the thyroid hormones. It is also thought to be connected to skin cancer, microbial imbalances, muscle fatigue, and weakness, impacts the endocrine system, and may contribute to allergies.

Found In:	Alternative/Solution:
Antibacterial soaps	Castile soap, essential oil-based hand sanitizers
Toothpastes	Natural, organic toothpaste
Mouthwash	Coconut oil pulling, triclosan-free essential oil mouthwashes
Household cleaners	Green, organic household cleaners

Perchloroethylene (PERC)

Similar to VOCs, perchloroethylene is found in clothes that have been dry-cleaned and shoe polish. Also known as tetrachloroethylene, PERC is a typical dry cleaning solution because it lifts stubborn spots and stains from clothing. To give you an idea of how powerful it is, it is a chemical often used in paint strippers.

One of the ironies of toxins is that they are inconsistently labeled when it comes to application and use. When PERC is used in paint strippers, it is advised to use masks and gloves, whereas when added to dry cleaning products, it doesn't. However, this only highlights our ignorance of what actually goes into products, and we must use every resource to educate ourselves and make mindful choices.

However, the consequence may be considered more severe as even the smallest drop is highly toxic and has been linked to liver and kidney dysfunction, dizziness, neurological effects, cancers, disruptions to the menstrual cycle, and congenital disabilities (and sometimes miscarriages).

Found In:	Alternative/Solution:
Dry cleaning products	Avoid clothing that requires dry cleaning. Use wet-cleaning techniques and clean at home rather than sending products to the dry cleaners.
Shoe polish	Natural polishes made from nuts, pigments, coconut oil, and clay

Parabens

Parabens are added to millions of household items to increase their shelf life — this ranges from food to pharmaceuticals and everything in between. In the bathroom and laundry room, they are typically found in makeup, perfume, shampoos, conditioner, shaving products, and lotions. There are many varieties of parabens, most ending in 'paraben.' Common parabens include, methylparaben, ethylparaben, propylparaben, isopropylparaben, butylparaben, and isobutylparaben. Parabens are particularly dangerous for women as they disrupt hormones, impacting menstrual cycles, fertility, congenital disorders, and breast cancer. It can also trigger early puberty in young girls.

The self-care industry is beginning to wake up to the fact that parabens are dangerous, and we just don't want them in the products they sell — even major corporations are starting to carry natural product lines. Things like shampoo bars and clarifying soaps free from parabens and other pollutants (such as sulfites, formaldehyde, and dyes) are now available widely. Online stores such as carinaorganics.com and rockymountainsoap.com sell numerous products that are safe to use. Other places like Etsy and farmer's markets can also contain such products.

We must not keep quiet about the dangers of parabens and other toxins. We can make our voices heard through online social media posts, recommending this book to friends and family, and writing letters and emails to corporations to exclude these ingredients from their formulas. We can vote with our dollars every time we shop, and indeed, we do so every time we don't buy products with toxins and instead opt for natural, organic, and healthy alternatives. We can't depend on others for our health. We must take action and make lasting changes.

Found In:	Alternative/Solution:
Makeup	Natural, organic makeup
Perfume	Essential oils mixed with carrier oils
Shampoo/conditioner	Toxin-free, natural, and organic shampoos and conditioners
Lotion	Toxin-free, natural, and organic lotions
Shaving products	Toxin-free, natural, and organic shaving bars

Bleach

Bleach is a generic term referring to toxins that lighten or whiten clothing and other substances — two common bleaches are chlorine and peroxide. Because bleach is a cheap additive that gets many jobs done, it is added to hundreds of household cleaners. They are used to kill bacteria, viruses, mold, and algae.

Too much bleach can lead to eye and skin irritations, chlorine poisoning, and bronchospasms. The risks of side effects and consequences drastically increase when mixing chemical cleaners—for example, toilet bowl cleaner (which contains bleach) and ammonia. A scientific study highlighted the danger when it said, "A dangerous problem with bleach occurs if bleach is mixed with other household cleaners, especially toilet bowl cleaners, and ammonia. These mixtures result in the release of chlorine gas, an asphyxiant. When chlorine gas contacts moist tissues, such as eyes or lungs, hydrochloric acid (HCl) results. **This acid is a digestive molecule and damages tissue. It will cause damage to the airways, asphyxiation, and can result in death."** [2]

When I was a teenager, one of my chores was to wash the floor — and I prided myself in doing a good job. I would mix whatever cleaners were available, aka chemicals, not knowing how dangerous it was. There would be fumes and bubbles, and the floor would get clean. However, unbeknown to me, I may have been only one chemical away from making a deadly mixture!

Other dangerous combinations are bleach and vinegar (produces chlorine gas), multiple drain cleaners (produces toxic vapors and fumes), hydrogen peroxide and vinegar (produces peracetic acid), mildew stain removers and bleach (produces chlorine gas), and bleach and rubbing alcohol (produces chloroform).

Bleach can easily be substituted for safer options such as lemon essential oil, white vinegar, and 'A' rating oxygenated bleaches. There are also DIY options (see the bonus chapter) and green, natural, all-purpose cleaners readily available at large grocery chains.

Found In:	Alternative/Solution:
Household cleaners	White vinegar, lemon essential oil, oxygen-based bleach
Bleach	White vinegar

Formaldehyde*

Thus far, we have briefly mentioned formaldehyde, but let's take another quick look at it and how it can be found in your bathroom and laundry room products. It is found in things such as bathroom vanities, mops, shampoos, body wash, and hair gel. Formaldehyde can cause organ and respiratory failure, resulting in death, and with bathrooms and laundry rooms typically being very small rooms with many things packed into them, the risk of formaldehyde poisoning is real. Early signs of the formaldehyde irritating your systems are a burning sensation in the eyes, nose, and throat, along with chemical burns upon skin contact. People who have medical conditions such as asthma will find their symptoms magnified.

Personal care items are a great first place to begin your toxin-free life. Take a look at your various personal care items, and if they contain any of the following, then it is time to replace them! Look for:

- methylene glycol
- DMDM hydantoin
- imidazolidinyl urea
- Diazolidinyl urea
- quaternium 15
- Bronopol
- 5-bromo-5-nitro-1
- 3 dioxane and hydroxymethyl glycinate

Found In:	Alternative/Solution:
Mops	Wood handled mops, bamboo or cellulose cleaning cloths
Personal care item	Greener and natural equivalents
Modified/artificial wood products and resins (such as vanities)	Vanities made from real wood and stone countertops, seal exposed sides

Butylated Hydroxyanisole (BHA) & Butylated Hydroxytoluene (BHT)*

BHA and BHT are some of the many toxins found in intimate and personal care products. In fact, it is often found in many of the products already discussed in this chapter! It is linked to various neurological problems, is an endocrine disruptor, and can cause reproductive issues.

Found In:	Alternative/Solution:
Makeup	Natural, organic makeup
Perfume	Essential oils
Shampoo/conditioner	Toxin-free, natural, and organic shampoos and conditioners
Lotion	Toxin-free, natural, and organic lotions
Shaving products	Toxin-free, natural, and organic shaving bars
Deodorant/antiperspirant	Deodorant rocks, all-natural deodorants
Toilet bowl cleaner	DIY toilet bowl cleaner (see the bonus section for a recipe!), pumice cleaning stones

On top of BHAs, BHTs, and VOCs found in antiperspirants, it's important to note that antiperspirants have many different chemicals, and one that prevents you from sweating, aluminum. While studies are not conclusive about whether the aluminum in them causes cancer, aluminum is linked to bone disease, kidney disease, and memory disorders and should absolutely be avoided. It may take time to find a non-toxic deodorant that works for you, but the experimentation will be well worth it for your long-term health.

Sodium Lauryl Sulfate (SLS)

When products are both oil and water-based, they often contain SLS or a similar product to combine them (oil and water don't mix!), making it a surfactant. It is also a foaming agent. It is found in self-care products (makeup, cream, lotions, bubble bath soap, hand soaps, hair care, toothpaste, etc.) and in cleaning products (grease removers, soaps, all-purpose cleaners, etc.).

And, if that wasn't enough, it is also permitted in food! The FDA allows it to make marshmallows fluffier, fruit juices, and dried eggs.

Many people report that SLS is relatively safe as it only causes rashes and skin irritations when used in excess. However, considering that it is used in many lotions and food products — two places where we do not want to cause rashes are our skin and internal organs! It is best to stay away from all products that use SLS.

Found In:	Alternative/Solution:
Self-care and cleaning products	Natural, green products without toxins. Many DIY products do not call for SLS to make it an effective alternative.

Sodium Hydroxide (Lye)

Sodium hydroxide is a colorless, odorless chemical that is corrosive and can cause significant damage if inhaled or touched. It is often found in soaps and cleaners, including bar soaps, drain cleaners, and detergents. Lye is used in the bar soap-making process but do not have any lye in them when complete and, therefore, safe to use. If making soap, safe soap-making precautions must be taken, including wearing gloves and goggles.

It is found in its true form in drain cleaners and multipurpose cleaners. Side effects of exposure to sodium hydroxide include burns, vomiting, fatigue, diarrhea, and damage to the throat, eyes, nose, and lungs. Long-term damage includes permanent damage to the lungs and digestive system.

Found In:	Alternative/Solution:
Cleaning products	White vinegar, lemon essential oil
Drain cleaner	Baking soda and white vinegar

HAIR DYE

"I know a lot about dyes and dye stuffs in the textile industry. We would never dream of using this on textiles. Primitive, archaic, all these things come to mind. Why do they persist on putting it on human heads?" says David Lewis, an emeritus professor at the University of Leeds, referring to the most common dyes people use.[4]

Dyes are filled with toxins linked to bladder and breast cancer, asthma, severe acne and other skin conditions, and liver and blood toxicity. When it comes to toxins, some people are under the impression that having exposure to them only increases their risk of the side effects they produce by marginal amounts; however, that is not the case. Chemical hair dyes increase women's risk of breast cancer by 23%, which is only one of the many potential side effects dyes can cause.[5] There are three common ingredients in dyes:

- *Ammonia* — breaks up the hair proteins for the dye to reach the hair shafts.
- *P-phenylenediamine* — the foundational coloring agent formed from petroleum (it is formed from coal tar).
- *Hydrogen peroxide* — Bleaches the hair so that the new color appears correctly. The percentage ratio is the key to determining the safety of it. A 3% hydrogen peroxide is a mild antiseptic and is safe to use on cuts. The percentage in hair dyes is much higher, and when combined with other chemicals, it becomes toxic, leading to rashes, allergies, and hair damage.

Hair dyes are incredibly toxic because they are applied very close to the scalp, allowing it to absorb the chemicals into the bloodstream. The FDA does not regulate most dyes used by hair stylists, therefore making it difficult to know what chemicals are in them in addition to the three listed above.

Today, there are chemical-free dyes such as Radico — which is henna plus the addition of herbs such as indigo that give it different shades of red all the way up to black, depending on the ratio — and more hair stylists are beginning to allow customers to bring their own dye (there is also always the option to do it yourself at home!).

BLACK HENNA

Henna is a type of body decoration and art that stains the skin and tends to be very intricate and patterned; it is often done on the hands, arms, and feet. It is used in many cultures to celebrate weddings, religious holidays, and birthdays. Black henna is a combination of henna and black hair dye that is laced with

P-phenylenediamine. This highly toxic chemical can result in chemical burning and long-term consequences such as cancer, asthma, and kidney damage.

Natural henna or mehndi, which is henna that is made from the Lawsonia Inermis plant, is very safe and is only a combination of the dried plant, lemon juice, sugar, essential oil, and tea (recipes will vary). It leaves an orange/dark red/brown/cherry black stain (never a true black color) on the skin that continues to darken for up to forty-eight hours of application.

JAGUA

Jagua, a Genipa Americana fruit found in South America, was often used by Native tribes for body decoration. Despite its high nutritional value, the fruit is most frequently harvested and utilized as a blue-black dye. Like henna, jagua is a temporary stain that lasts approximately ten to fourteen days. However, unlike henna, it dries flat, and the dark blue-black color makes it look more like an authentic tattoo rather than the decorative effect henna has.

FEMININE HYGIENE PRODUCTS

Feminine hygiene products are a collective term for pads (sanitary napkins), tampons, sprays, washes, powders, and wipes, some necessary and others not. Every woman for a few decades of their life has their period and regularly needs products to clean up after themselves.

Many of the toxins found in hygiene products are endocrine disruptors, meaning they can affect hormones, reproductive systems, thyroid, and ovaries. These aren't things you can take

DETOX: THE BATHROOM & LAUNDRY ROOM

risks with. You deserve to feel the absolute best you can — we live in a day and age when medical care has never been so good, yet we don't fix the root of the problem: the toxins found in and on millions of everyday household items.

The vagina and vulva are very absorbent areas with a multitude of blood vessels and arteries that can transport the chemicals found in feminine hygiene products directly into the bloodstream. These chemicals (whether from the absorbent materials, plastic liners, or fragrances) are endocrine-disrupting, with many being VOCs. Common chemicals found in feminine products include n-heptane, carbon tetrachloride, n-nonane, n-hexane, 1,4-dioxane, α-pinene, benzene, toluene, styrene, limonene, and 1,2,4-trimethylbenzene. There are up to forty-five different VOCs in a single hygiene product, and the number of VOCs does not vary for products labeled as 'for sensitive skin' or if they contain 'natural' products![3]

Periods should be pain-free, without intense cravings and excessive bloating — and this can be done to a large extent by removing toxins from your food and home. Your period shouldn't cause you to miss events and work, to have crazy hormones, and to feel depressed — and you can change how future periods are. In my own life, I have noticed a massive difference in my periods and no longer dread them; yes, they are still not always convenient or perfect, but I am able to go about my daily business and work without a second thought or pain.

Once your period is over for the month, you shouldn't have to worry about vaginal conditions. Still, unfortunately, bacterial and yeast irritations or infections are all too common, as are dryness or itchiness. Other conditions, such as pelvic infections and cervical cancer, remain a constant threat when we don't remove toxins from the products we use.

Right now, one easy thing to do is stop using feminine washes, which are a cocktail of unnecessary chemicals and fragrances. They disrupt the natural bacteria and cause infections, allergic reactions, and irritation. Opt for cleaning daily with warm water only.

Found In:	Alternative/Solution:
Pads (sanitary napkins)	Cloth pads, cotton pads that are compostable
Tampons	Menstrual cups, and discs

It's important to note that many of the same chemicals found in pads can also be found in diapers for babies and adults. Babies essentially live in diapers on average between 18-30 months! How often do we think that we are constantly exposing them to chemicals? I admit it was not a thought that crossed my mind. Also, each child produces approximately a mountain's worth of diapers that never break down and go away. That is why I switched my third child to cloth diapers; we already had two diaper mountains out there and didn't want another! It's time to choose better options for them and the planet.

Found In:	Alternative/Solution:
Diapers	Cloth diapers, biodegradable disposable diapers

TOILET PAPER

Unfortunately, this was one of the last things to make it to my list. Oddly enough, I didn't think a light paper material would contain a plethora of chemicals. In hindsight, it should have been one of the first things I thought of, considering how often it is used on a daily basis and on such delicate body parts. Toilet paper contains PFAs, chlorine, dioxins, formaldehyde, petroleum-based compounds, and in some instances, fragrances and dyes. These chemicals not only affect your health, but also cause water pollution.

Most toilet paper brands found in stores are guilty of containing at least some of these toxins. Brands, such as Caboo, are toxin-free and are made from sustainable bamboo.

Finding a suitable toilet paper that is affordable might not be a solution for everyone. A cheaper and more eco-friendly solution would be to clean with water (more on that below) and gently pat dry with toilet paper or designated cloth sheets. This way, you avoid vigorous rubbing, which increases your exposure to the chemicals embedded in the toilet paper.

Found In:	Alternative/Solution:
Toilet Paper	Cloth sheets and a wet bag, non-toxic toilet paper

GOOD HYGIENE PRACTICES

Now that we've discussed possible chemicals and mold issues that may be lurking in your bathroom. Let's discuss the risks of poor hygiene practices. Handwashing after using the toilet may seem like common sense to most, but it is overlooked by some. It is absolutely necessary to avoid spreading germs and risk getting yourself and others sick. Just a tiny amount of feces can contain a trillion germs! Door knobs, handles, handrails, computers, and anything touched can be contaminated. This unsanitary practice leads to gastrointestinal problems, diarrhea, cases of flu, eye infections, and so much more.

It is also vital to clean one's behind properly after using the toilet, which is often neglected in the Western world. Streptococcus and other bacteria can be present in the private regions and can lead to severe illnesses if not cleaned properly. Gentle cleaning with water and drying after using the toilet will help reduce infections, itchiness, and odor. Install a bidet, or use a *lota,* the South Asian name for a watering can, kept in the bathroom for hygiene purposes. Then, washing hands with soap and water will help reduce the risk of spreading unwanted germs.

Top Five Things to Do Today:

- ❖ Replace shampoos, conditioners, and body washes with green, natural, and organic options
- ❖ Replace pads with fragrance-free, fully compostable, and organic pads, and tampons with menstrual cups or discs
- ❖ Replace laundry detergents with all-natural or DIY alternatives (see bonus chapter!)
- ❖ Replace dryer sheets with wool dryer balls
- ❖ Use natural hair dye and henna as opposed to their chemical alternatives

CONCLUSION

Toxins can be found everywhere in our laundry room and bathrooms. We could cover thousands of different products in these rooms that are filled with various chemicals, toxins, and heavy metals. Removing the toxins from these rooms can be overwhelming; however, start with just one item per week or per month and slowly begin switching the items you use the most frequently. Change starts with you, and those changes will have a lasting positive effect on your health and will bring many benefits to the overall health of your home and family.

[1] Rather than refer you back to Chapter One for more information about a specific chemical or toxin, I noted this with an asterisk (*). Therefore, when you see the symbol, know that when you need more information (or just a refresher) about it, please jump back to chapter one.

5

DETOX: THE BEDROOM & OFFICE

What's the danger of sleeping in a room riddled with toxins like VOCs and synthetic fragrances? The answer comes from Marilee Nelson, cofounder of the natural cleaning line Branch Basics. "The body never gets the chance to rest, recover, and recuperate," she says, "because it's busy detoxing these chemicals."

Unbeknown to many, there are chemicals in bedrooms, from the mattress you lay on to the comforter that covers you; chemicals encompass you as you sleep. When you go to work, the toxins in the paint on the walls surrounding you, the cushions in the chair you sit on, and the carpet you rest your feet on continue to envelop you. While not visible to the human eye, your hormones are slowly set out of balance, your risk for cancer increases, and your organs can be damaged. But it's time to reverse all that, so let's detox the bedroom and office!

TOXINS PRESENT

Polybrominated Diphenyl Ethers (PBDE)*

PBDEs are flame retardants, which slow the ignition and spread of fires. However, when fires do occur, the fumes they produce are so toxic that they contribute to deaths related to fires. In the bedroom and office, they are found in the foam cushions of furniture, bed linens, mattresses, and curtains — all this can cause or contribute to brain damage, nerve damage, thyroid disruption, and developmental toxicity. The last condition mentioned is nothing to joke about; babies and toddlers have three to nine times more PBDE in their systems than adults.

Some businesses, such as IKEA, have been actively phasing out PBDEs. However, before purchasing items that could contain flame retardants, do a quick Google search to ensure you're not accidentally buying products with toxins.

Found In:	Alternative/Solution:
Mattress	Organic mattresses
Throw pillows and furniture cushions	Organic pillows, cushions that state that they contain no added flame retardant chemicals
Bed linens/sheets	Natural fiber sheets (such as 100% bamboo or cotton without synthetic dyes)

With the rise of the Internet in the last few years, it is much easier to find all-natural, organic mattresses that won't affect your health — and won't break the bank! Our top favorite mattress brands are:

1. Birch – slightly firm yet provides comfort and support for the whole body. Birch mattresses are affordable and use cotton, latex, and wool in their makeup.

2. Brentwood Home — the most affordable option on this list, Brentwood mattresses are natural, good for your health, and come in various sizes.
3. Awara — similar to Birch mattresses, Awara mattresses are slightly less firm and somewhat more affordable.
4. Silk & Snow - better materials. And different types in varying yet more affordable price ranges. I've personally switched my mattress to one of theirs.

When you sleep, your body goes to work repairing itself. Many of us probably remember our mothers telling us not to eat before we go to bed because when our bodies digest food, it takes away from it, rejuvenating and cleaning up damaged or destroyed cells. From gut health to optimal brain functionality, our sleeping bodies do an immense amount of work so we can have the strength and durability to do the tasks set before us.

When we sleep on toxic mattresses, our body can't devote itself entirely to the restoration it needs as it has to focus some of its energy on detoxing the chemicals. The answer is always a mattress void of fire retardants, VOCs, heavy metals, and vinyl.

An Interim Solution

If a new mattress is not yet in your budget, you can mitigate some of the toxins by adding an all-organic, toxin-free mattress protector and bed linens. 100% organic cotton sheets — readily available at very affordable prices — are free from pesticides and herbicides. Many regular cotton products are bleached and dyed, so stick to organic sheets that use only natural dyes if they contain patterns or designs.

Phthalates*

The higher the levels of phthalates in your urine, the more likely you are to die of heart disease — a startling and frightening thought! It has also been linked to asthma, ADHD, breast cancer, and neurodevelopmental issues.

My bedroom is my oasis, and while it's not a spa, it does contain some of my favorite things that help me relax, including more than one fragrance candle — unfortunately, today, many of these now contain phthalates. Alternatives to them are essential oil diffusers or candles scented with essential oils.

Aromatherapy, the practice of diffusing essential oils, has been used for hundreds of years (as far back as ancient China, India, and Egypt) to stimulate the brain into relaxing, relieve pain and anxiety, and improve mood. Some people also use it to help them sleep.

Essential oils can be used in aromatherapy as follows:

- Chamomile – reduces stress and nervous tension
- Clary sage – relaxation, improves memory and concentration, reduces blood pressure, decreases period pain
- Eucalyptus – clears sinuses, reduces joint pain
- Geranium – balances hormones, reduce fluid retention
- Ginger – reduces nausea
- Lavender – aids sleep
- Lemon – improves mood, helps concentration
- Lemongrass – decreases stress/worry
- Peppermint – reduces headaches, increases alertness
- Roman Chamomile – reduces stress and nervous tension

❖ Rosemary – increases focus, reduces tension

Outside of aromatherapy, essential oils can be used to treat many conditions and are an excellent starting point to move away from toxic medications. Just one drop of essential oils can have anywhere from 250 to 800 different elements that work to improve and rejuvenate your body! Adding a diffuser to your bedroom can help you sleep or keep you alert and focused in your office. If using in the home, ensure the essential oils are safe for your pets.

Found In:	Alternative/Solution:
Candles	Beeswax or soy wax candles scented with essential oils
Air fresheners	Air diffusers and essential oils
Yoga mats	Organic cotton, jute, natural rubber, or cork

Volatile Organic Compounds (VOC)*

By now, VOCs should not be a surprise to you – they are found in every room of the home! In the bedroom and office, they are often found in wall paint, vinyl flooring (especially vinyl rolls and sheets), and some engineered wood. It is linked to eye, nose, and throat irritations, liver and kidney damage, and various cancers.

When you open a can of paint, and a wave of fumes hits you, that is a strong indication that your paint contains VOCs. Lead paint test kits can be purchased at most major big-box hardware or specialty paint stores. When used correctly, most kits have about a 95% accuracy rate, and buying two or three different brands will give a very accurate result. When shopping for new paints, be sure to get zero-VOC paint rather than low-VOC paint.

Found In:	Alternative/Solution:
Vinyl flooring	Real wood flooring, real linoleum, tile flooring, cork flooring, or look for zero-VOC vinyl planks
Lead paint	Zero-VOC paint
Engineered wood	Real wood furniture, or seal the exposed edges with shellac

Formaldehyde

There is something incredibly satisfying about having wrinkle-free bed sheets and covers — but are they really attractive when you know that they are laced in formaldehyde so that they retain their wrinkle-free status?

Formaldehyde is frequently found in engineered wood (also known as pressed wood or particle board). Today, millions of pieces of furniture are made with this artificial wood, and formaldehyde is just one of the chemicals found in them. Replacing this type of furniture can be costly, but begin by replacing just one small piece of furniture — such as a side table or sideboard — and then sell it, allowing yourself to recoup some of the cost to replace the item. Last year, a friend replaced her engineered wood bookcases with two oak bookcases she found on Facebook Marketplace for $150; with a little bit of elbow grease and a new coat of natural stain, she had a set of bookcases that gets many more compliments than her old bookcases got (which by the way she sold for $100!). Estate sales, thrift stores, Facebook Marketplace, and Craig's List are great places to shop for real wood furniture.

When you are in the process of switching out your furniture, consider having the pressed wood pieces scattered throughout the home so as not to concentrate the toxins they left off in one area. Toxins are also found in particle board paneling, which can be replaced with real wood paneling, or particle board paneling that doesn't contain a formaldehyde resin (you'll have to consult your local hardware store for this) or one with a soy-based adhesive.

A newer, somewhat effective option is to apply a seal over the unsealed particle board products and other products that contain VOCs.

If these options don't work for you, from now on, be more mindful of what furniture you bring into your home.

Found In:	Alternative/Solution:
Engineered wood	Real wood furniture
Particle board and paneling	Read wood paneling, boards with no formaldehyde resin or soy-based adhesives

Perfluoroalkyl and Polyfluoroalkyl Substances (PFAS)*

Forever chemicals are often found in the cloth materials of bedrooms and offices: clothing, curtains, upholstery, and water-resistant fabrics (such as on office chairs). These toxins decrease fertility, developmental delays, and low birth weights for babies. It can also cause high blood pressure, disrupt hormones, increase cholesterol, and damage the immune system.

Several years ago, I used to own a set of curtains that produced a terrible odor once the sun shone on them. While I'm unsure what chemicals they were projecting, they were most undoubtedly toxic. Be very careful about every product you add to your home — including window coverings!

Found In:	Alternative/Solution:
Clothing, curtains, furniture	Natural fiber clothing and materials

TECHNOLOGY

EMFs and Blue Light

When the electric and magnetic fields are combined, they are referred to as electromagnetic fields, commonly abbreviated as EMFs. This field has two main categories: low and high energy. Today, we are continually exposed to one particular low-energy EMF: blue light. Blue light EMFs have immediate effects on our eye health: eye strain and fatigue, and crow lines around the eyes. A significant issue unrelated to the eyes is that it negatively impacts our circadian rhythm as it prevents the body from producing melatonin, a hormone that helps us go to sleep. Longer-term effects include dry eyes and overall deterioration of the eye. Digital screens (such as phones and laptops) popularly use LED lighting as it takes very little energy to produce and is durable. However, as companies begin to understand the harmful effects of blue light, many blue light filters are available, and many eyeglass prescriptions also have a blue light filtration in the lens. Eye comfort settings can also be found on newer phones, which reduce blue light and show warmer colors that can help protect your eyes. Take advantage of filters and eye comfort settings to give your eyes relief.

DETOXING WHILE YOU WORK AND SLEEP

Removing the extra chemicals from your home is always a good idea. As you transition your home, there are several ways you can continue to detox without it being obvious or expensive.

1. Open a window. Fresh air is always a good idea as it helps to remove toxins from the air and makes the home smell fresh and inviting. Since indoor air pollution ranges from three to five times higher than outdoor air pollution, it's always a good idea to prop open a window! During colder months, there are air filtration systems that can help purify the air — but don't forget to change out the furnace filters regularly!

2. Add plants. Plants are known to be natural filtration systems, drawing on the CO2 and formaldehyde in the air to produce clean oxygen. Palm trees, Boston ferns, rubber plants, and aloe vera are some of the best detoxification plants. Just be sure the plant (such as lilies) isn't toxic for your pets.

3. Removing electronic devices from the room. Turning off electronic devices helps to reduce radiation transmission – which makes it longer for people to fall asleep and stay in a deep sleep. It also reduces light pollution, which can affect your sleep. Try refraining from using devices too close to bedtime in order to get good quality sleep, which is needed to detox your body from the day's stresses and toxins.

CLOTHING

In the previous section, clothing was mentioned several times as toxins are found in many types. An acquaintance recently got into a frenzy of buying clothes from Shein, a very cheap clothing website. She could buy a sweater, dress, or top for just a few dollars, and she didn't mind if it fell apart after a few months of wear; it was cheap enough to easily replace. One evening, she made a casserole for her family, one that she had made several times, and as usual, after fifty minutes, she pulled it out of the oven, piping hot and ready to be eaten. However, on this particular evening, she was wearing a new sweater from Shein, and as quickly as she pulled the dish from the oven, she threw it on the stovetop, gasping at the burning sensation in her arm. White with pain, she pulled up her sleeve to see that the threads in the sweater had melted onto her skin — the pan hadn't even touched her arm, but in a few split seconds, the materials used in the sweater were weak enough to melt and cause third degree burns on her arm! These toxins found in the fabric of her sweater caused burns in just a few seconds when she got too close to heat — think about what could have happened if she was straightening or curling her hair, ironing, or was frying greasy food that could have splattered onto her sweater? Fast fashion comes at a price, and it could have been her life. Companies specializing in fast fashion are often involved in cruel labor practices — child labor, forced enslavement, or unreasonable hours. They are interested in their bottom line and not about the environment or people's health — and most certainly not about the toxins in their products. Add to that, they are often made in far-away lands with few safety regulations and then expend millions of tons of toxins into the air and sea to transport the goods.

Sustainable clothing

Many women, at times myself included, love shopping for new clothing. The thrill of finding a shirt or tunic that matches your personality, that fits well, and brings a smile to your face is worth the search. Learning to shop sustainably can ensure our bodies aren't suffering from our desire to be stylish while also protecting women and children who work in terrible conditions to produce cheap clothes.

One of the arguments often used by proponents of fast fashion is that it is much more affordable than sustainable clothing. However, rather than buying cheap items, look for items you can easily wear from season to season. Find items that will last beyond a few washes, won't pill or snag, and have good structure and support — you're looking for quality over quantity.

Other ways to practice clothing sustainability:

> ❖ Shop second-hand (including your sister's and friend's closets!). Consignment shops often have higher-end pieces at discount prices.
> ❖ Only buy clothes you love – not because it is on sale or because it is just 'okay.'
> ❖ Shop locally and avoid online mass retailers.
> ❖ Shop sustainable brands that focus on sustainability.
> ❖ Donate, reuse, recycle, or sell unused clothing.
> ❖ Hold a clothing exchange party with friends where everyone brings their unwanted clothing, and it is a free-for-all event.

Some fabrics contain toxins in them. Fabrics to avoid are polyester, nylon, spandex, and acrylic. Look for 100% cotton, silk, wool, bamboo, or flax products. Or look for the OEKO-TEX certification that indicates that the clothing is free from harmful substances.

CONCLUSION

Your bedroom should be a safe haven, free from toxins, and between it and your office, you spend over half your day in these rooms. It only makes sense that they are a priority in your toxin-free journey. The same goes for your children: each room in your home should be safe, especially children's bedrooms, as they spend hours every day sleeping there.

Five Things You Can Do Today:

❖ Open a window! Air flow is critical to detoxing the home.

❖ Buy a plant, or find one in a Buy Nothing Group to help filter and purify the air.

❖ Get rid of clothing you don't wear. Some may contain toxins, and there is no point in holding on to them unnecessarily.

❖ Replace bed sheets and linens with 100% organic cotton sheets. Ensure that if they have prints, they only use natural dye.

❖ Purchase a diffuser and essential oils to combat the toxins in the office, improve your concentration, and detox the room.

6

DETOX: THE LIVING ROOM & PLAYROOM

Did you know that the average American now spends approximately 90% of their time indoors—and that the concentration of some pollutants and toxins is two to five times higher indoors than outdoors? That means that the average American is spending more time in a highly polluted environment!

Many of these toxins can be found in the living room and playroom. As we go through these two rooms, we'll explore how they came into the home and what you can do to mitigate and remove them.

Asbestos*

Many people are aware that asbestos is not good for your health. However, if they are left undisturbed, their dangers are not as drastic as when bathed in them. I was aware of this since I remembered an incident at my elementary school where the asbestos was disturbed, and we weren't able to enter until it was cleaned up. Still, I never realized how dangerous it was until an acquaintance, Jude, got sick. Jude and her husband had purchased an older home with the intention of slowly renovating it while living there with their three kids. Since they were ambitious and handy, they fully intended to do it all themselves — beginning with their kitchen and living room. Because they both worked during the day, the process dragged on, and often, they went to bed with dust particles still floating in the air as they drifted off to sleep. A few months into the renovations, Jude began to feel tired, chalking it up to the stress and extra work the renovations were causing. Three months later, she was put on medical leave and struggled to get out of bed — she lost her appetite and struggled with each breath. The cause? Asbestos had been found in the ceiling, and when they had scrapped the popcorn ceiling off, the asbestos particles went wild. It had a devastating consequence on her health. Three years have passed, the flip house project was abandoned, and Jude is still on medical leave. She has lost over fifty pounds, but in recent months, it seems as though she may finally be turning a page in her health. Her appetite seems to be returning, although she still has a long way to go. The toxins in that home nearly cost her life: we don't realize how devastating toxins can be until they hit home.

Asbestos can be very dangerous, and homes built before the mid-1980s often contain them. It can be found in everything from window caulking and glazing to HVAC duct insulation. Plaster (drywall and putty), vinyl flooring, 'the red embers' in gas-lit fireplaces, and textured paint have all been found to contain asbestos. It is linked to serious health effects such as pleural plaques, asbestosis, lung cancer, and mesothelioma.

If you suspect asbestos may be in the structure of your home, the first course of action is to call a certified professional in asbestos identification and removal. Asbestos is not something you want to mess around with, and hiring professionals is the best way to keep your and your family's health safe. If you don't have the resources to remove asbestos from your home, the next best is to do nothing. Leaving asbestos undisturbed can keep it 'dormant,' which is much safer than any DIY attempt that instantly releases thousands of asbestos toxins into the air.

Found In:	Alternative/Solution:
Structural framework in homes built before 1980.	Live in a home newer than 1980. If the home is older, consider getting it tested and then decide from there what course of action you'll follow.

Volatile Organic Compounds (VOC)*

By now, you are very familiar with VOCs and can guess how they are found in the living room and playroom: wall paint, pressed wood furniture, and vinyl flooring. Early symptoms of exposure include headaches, nausea, allergic reactions, and fatigue. Long-term exposure can cause eye, nose, and throat irritation, liver, central nervous system, kidney damage, and some types of cancer.

A more extreme solution to removing VOCs from your home is replacing your vinyl floors with real wood flooring, real linoleum, tiles, cork, or zero-VOC vinyl planks. This is an expensive and large project to undertake, so I recommend that until it is practical to undertake this, focus on more minor improvements and projects in the living room and playroom!

Found In:	Alternative/Solution:
Wall paints	Test the walls for VOC paints. If your walls have paint that is high in volume of VOCs, repaint it with a VOC-free paint. Big-name brands such as Behr and Sherwin-Williams both carry zero-VOC paints; there are also many smaller and local brands that carry zero-VOC paints.
Flooring	Tile, cork, real linoleum, natural hardwood, or other appropriate flooring

Formaldehyde

In the living room and playroom, formaldehyde is found in the pressed wood of the bookcases, toy boxes, cabinets, and other pressed wood items. On the walls, it is found in particle boards and paneling, and in the walls, it is found in foam insulation. The first signs of formaldehyde poisoning are watery eyes, headaches, nausea, allergies, and coughing. Long term, it is linked to asthma, breast cancer, obesity, Type-2 diabetes, neurodevelopmental issues, and male fertility issues; it also increases people's risk of developing ADHD.

I recommend you change pressed wood furniture for real wood alternatives. If you can't, apply soy-based adhesives made with soy flour and a curing agent or a product called SafeCoat to trap the formaldehyde (it also works for trapping VOCs).

An Interim Solution

In the meantime, ensure that pressed wood is out of reach for small children who are likelier to touch and eat things they should not.

Found In:	Alternative/Solution:
Furniture	Replace with real wood furniture or seal with SafeCoat

Lead

As mentioned in previous chapters, lead is often found in old paint made or applied before 1978. It can cause cognitive issues, decreased IQ, behavioral issues, reproductive system damage, abdominal pains, increased blood pressure, and anemia. Paint that contains lead becomes dangerous when it chips, fumes, or peels.

Dealing With Lead and Removing It

Where do people paint? Turns out, just about everywhere. The following surfaces are common places that people paint — and not always areas you'd remember to check and sand completely before applying a new coat of 'clean' paint:

- Doors - the interior spaces between the jam often forget to be painted, and it may still be exposing lead paint
- Stairs - the side treads are not repainted frequently
- Windowsills - because windows often are a damp area, layers of paint peel and can cause lead to be exposed
- Porches - rain and snow will chip away at the paint and expose lead paint.

Part One

Step One: Evaluating Paint

If you suspect lead paint (or any other type of toxic paint), run a test to appraise the paint if it contains toxins. Test different areas of the wall — top of the wall, bottom, middle, etc.

Step 2: Plan a Course of Action

If lead is detected, you'll want to pack up an overnight bag and find a safe place to live for a few weeks as you get it removed and painted over. Depending on either option, you'll need a place for at least a few weeks and, at the most, a few months. It is crucial that the paint is taken care of as it is especially dangerous for pregnant women and babies, children, and pets.

Once you've established that your walls contain toxins, you'll be able to decide whether or not this is a job you can do yourself or if it requires a professional. If you hire a professional (which I recommend you do to protect your safety), then stop the process here; if not, continue through steps three to seven. Throughout the process, remember to wear waterproof gloves and a mask.

Part Two:

Step 3: Clean the Area

Whether the toxic area is inside or outside, it should be cleaned. Lay down tarps to prevent floors and soil (the ground outside) from becoming saturated with the toxic paint. If the area is indoors, wipe it down with a damp cloth; if it's outside, hose it down with a pressure washer.

Step 4: Remove Paint

If the area is peeling or chipping, removing it before applying a fresh coat is essential. Use a scraper to scrape off all the loose areas, and then use some sandpaper to smooth the edges to prevent further peeling and for a smooth coat of paint.

Step 5: Paint!

Using a non-lead and non-VOC paint, apply a coat of paint to the walls — doing at least two coats is recommended.

Step 6: Clean Up

Once you have completed the repainting, it's time to finish things up by tidying the area. Fold the tarp towards the center so as not to spill any toxic paint chips on the ground.

Step 7: Discard Trash

Your first thought may be to throw the tarp in the garbage, but instead, it should be trashed at a toxic waste center.

Talcum Powder

Talcum powder is a toxin not yet discussed in this book. So, what is it? Talc is a mineral found in the earth's crust and is mined, often alongside asbestos and other toxic chemicals. After it is mined, it is crushed and mixed with silica and a little water. It is an absorbent often used in baby and feminine hygiene products to absorb liquids and moisture. It is also found in makeup, powders, soaps, chewing gum, rice, and candy.

Too much talc can lead to talc poisoning; signs of this include fatigue, blisters, vomiting, diarrhea, and weakness. More severe symptoms include fainting, coma, seizures, ovarian cancer, mesothelioma (a rare but severe type of cancer), lung damage, and dried mucus membranes.

Today, there are many alternatives to using talcum powder, including tapioca powder, corn starch, or arrowroot powder. Even big-name companies are beginning to come up with alternatives, such as Burt's Bees Baby Dusting Powder.

Found In:	Alternative/Solution:
Baby powder	All natural, organic, healthy baby powders that are talc-free
Makeup	Natural and organic powders that are talc-free
Soaps	Talc-free soaps
Gum	Avoid it altogether
Rice	Rice (check the label that it only has rice as an ingredient)
Candy	Dried fruit, organic/healthy alternatives

TOXIC TOYS

The issue of toxic toys has become a growing concern for parents and caregivers alike. Toxic toys refer to playthings that contain harmful substances or pose a risk to children's wellbeing. These hazardous materials can include lead, phthalates, bisphenol A (BPA), and other chemicals linked to developmental issues, hormone disruption, and even cancer. With childhood cancer on the rise, this could possibly be connected to the toys they play with.

The consequences of exposing children to toxic toys can be severe. Young minds are especially vulnerable during their formative years, so we must take every precaution necessary to ensure their safety. As responsible adults, it is our duty to stay informed about the potential dangers lurking in the products we bring into our homes.

Thankfully, awareness surrounding this issue has grown significantly in recent years. Governments worldwide have implemented stricter regulations on toy manufacturing processes and materials used. Additionally, consumer advocacy groups have been instrumental in raising awareness about specific brands or products that may pose a risk.

DETOX: THE LIVING ROOM & PLAYROOM

However, despite these efforts, there is still work to be done. Parents and caregivers need to remain vigilant when selecting toys for their children. Reading product labels carefully for any warnings or certifications can help identify potential hazards.

Furthermore, staying informed about recalls or safety alerts issued by regulatory bodies such as the Consumer Product Safety Commission (CPSC) can provide valuable insights into potentially dangerous products already on the market.

Ultimately, protecting our children from toxic toys requires a collective effort from manufacturers, regulators, advocacy groups, and consumers alike. By working together towards stricter regulations and promoting awareness surrounding this issue, we can ensure a safer environment for our little ones to learn and play in without compromising their health or well-being. There is one category of toys that is particularly concerning: plastic toys.

PLASTIC TOYS

When you walk down the toy aisle at your favorite big-box store, you'll quickly notice a common theme among them: bright, colorful plastic toys. Very seldom will you see all-wood toys painted with natural dyes and paints. Now, walk into your child's playroom and watch them play with their toys. Children are in constant contact with toys, playing with them and often putting them in their mouths.

Many toys today contain plasticizers, flame retardants, VOCs, fragrances, phthalates, and so much more. A professor at the Technical Institute of Denmark stated the dangers — and the solution to these toxic chemicals: "Out of 419 chemicals found in hard, soft, and foam plastic materials used in children toys, we identified 126 substances that can potentially harm children's health either via cancer or non-cancer effects, including 31 plasticizers, 18 flame retardants, and 8 fragrances. Being harmful in our study means that for these chemicals, estimated exposure doses exceed regulatory Reference Doses (RfD) or cancer risks exceed regulatory risk thresholds. These substances should be prioritized for phase-out in toy materials and replaced with safer and more sustainable alternatives." [1]

Since toys are not meant for consumption, the regulations surrounding them are much lower than food. With the average child in America and the Western world having over forty pounds of plastic and toxin-containing toys, the risk to children is worth considering. Because of all the toxins found in these toys, children are at higher risk for asthma, developing ADHD, obesity, type-2 diabetes, neurodevelopmental conditions, and nerve and brain damage.

A QUICK GUIDE TO GOOD TOYS

Since most plastics are out of the question, the focus will be on toxin-free toys such as BPA-free, VOC-free, fragrance-free, and phthalate-free.

1. Avoid cheap toys. From dollar stores to toys that come in kid's meals at fast food restaurants, the best thing to do is not to purchase them. Along with this, it is important to avoid most toys that are made in China as the quality control is limited there, and toxins are known to abound in them.

DETOX: THE LIVING ROOM & PLAYROOM

2. Avoid toys that are painted if made outside of the USA, Canada, or Western Europe, as paint may contain lead outside of these countries.

3. Look for toys that contain no glue or formaldehyde-free glue. It can be challenging to determine if the glue used is toxic (often, toys do not have product list ingredients). If you are unfamiliar with the company's practices, be cautious of buying products with glue.

4. Toys should only use natural paints and dyes to prevent lead contamination. Once again, you'll need to do some research on the company, but sometimes it is noted if the paint is natural.

5. Shop locally and on craft sites such as Etsy for unique toys that are natural and safe. Everything from cloth dolls to wooden toy trains can be found!

Toys (and other toxins) are often brought into the home through gifts or quick purchases when in a pinch. Having registries or specific lists can help weed out the potential for toxins to enter the home.

Removing toxins from your children's lives is just another way you take care of them. The symptoms of many childhood illnesses and conditions can be lessened or eradicated when toxins are removed from their toys and the home.

ARTIFICIAL FRAGRANCES

Artificial fragrances often contain petroleum-based ingredients that are harmful to your health — and often, the first symptoms of their toxicity begin by just walking into a room with them. A plug-in air freshener can have over twenty different VOCs!

I recently visited my dad and stepmom, and while walking through the rooms, I could sense the artificial fragrances that were being used were beginning to give me a headache. I asked them if we could change out all their plug-in fragrances, candles, and cleaners for non-toxic versions since we recently had a case of cancer in the family. Yes, I had done this many years ago, but I believe that because the clean products were not as common as they are now, it didn't stick. They agreed, so I figured the easiest way to make it stick for them was to take them shopping at a big-box store with sections labeled as "clean" where they were selling non-toxic products. We chose air fresheners and candles made with essential oils, and non-toxic cleaners. While some products might not have been the best in these sections, they certainly were better than the regular chemicals they were currently using and were a good starting point for them.

We all must start somewhere on our detoxification journey. For some, that means buying the best they can afford, but for others, that can mean they can buy the best products. As you begin, always do what is best for you and your budget. Any improvement, big or small, will be worth it.

FIVE THINGS YOU CAN DO TODAY:

❖ Add a ventilation system or fans to increase air circulation in the home. This will help remove toxins from the areas and bring in fresh air.

DETOX: THE LIVING ROOM & PLAYROOM

❖ Avoid talcum powder products; many all-natural, organic, and safe hygiene products are available today.

❖ Focus on buying wooden toys rather than plastic.

❖ Focus on quality items when shopping: this includes everything from food to furniture and toys.

❖ Start a list of items you want that are toxic-free — then, when asked about gifts or you want to purchase an item, you can refer back to the list to ensure that it is safe!

7

DETOX: BASEMENT, GARAGE, & OUTDOORS

Ariana scratched Duke, her Golden Retriever, between his ears. He lifted his head ever so slightly before resting it against his forepaws again, sighing deeply. Since the spring, he just hadn't been himself. Yes, he was starting to get older, but most Golden Retrievers his age were still energetic and didn't spend their days acting like they were lethargic and depressed.

Duke had been the family pet since he was eight weeks old. The kids loved him, and he did well with friends and guests who frequently came over. Everyone who knew him remarked about what a friendly dog he was: always happy with people and had a soft bark and a tail wag for those who gave him a quick pat. But that was now a thing of the past.

Ariana had taken Duke to the local vet twice, but nothing had been found. A few scans had been done — the vet thought it might be a tumor — but the scans came back fine. As did his blood work. His dog food had been switched to a healthier, more nutrient-dense alternative, but no change.

The doorbell rang. *Ah, finally!* Ariana thought. Her brother Adam was coming over for a few days from out of state. With a big grin on her face, she flung the door wide open and hugged her brother.

"It's been so long!" Ariana said. Adam stared back, scowling at her. "What's the matter?" she queried.

"I sneezed twice since pulling into your driveway," Adam said. "But your lawn looks amazing, whatever you're putting on it."

Ariana laughed. "That's so random," she said. "We hired a new maintenance company to do the lawn since we just don't have the time for it anymore. They are applying some mixture every few weeks on it."

Adam dropped his bags in the entryway and shut the door behind him. "Sis, you amaze me sometimes. You're so picky about the chemicals and garbage they put in things and ban so much from your house, and yet you allow some random company to spray it all over your yard. Bet you keep your windows open, too?"

Ariana froze. "Oh dear. That has never crossed my mind!"

That conversation was the start of yet another change in Ariana's home. She had been on a detoxification journey for many years — including what pesticides were used in the yard. When she hired the new lawn maintenance company, they had advertised that they were natural — but that was just a marketing word they used, and she didn't double-check that they didn't use any toxins. Unfortunately, they were using toxins on her grass. Her grass was green, but all the organisms and microbiology in it were mostly dead. Duke, who loved to play fetch in the yard and dig a few holes, also felt the effects of

DETOX: BASEMENT, GARAGE, & OUTDOORS

the sprays more than the family had. Ariana decided to cancel her contract with the lawn maintenance company. Today, the grass isn't quite as green and has some wildflowers now, but is still very healthy. The soil is thriving, but best of all, Duke has fully recovered and is back to his cheerful self.

Did you know that there are over 800 pesticides registered (and approved) for use in the USA? Unfortunately, even nature is subject to the toxic chemicals produced by humankind today. The number of toxins is amplified when we consider the types of things we store in our garages and spray in our yards.

The outdoor area is particularly subject to toxins when we consider all the pesticides, insecticides, and herbicides we spray to keep the bugs and weeds away. But whether a toxin is trapped in our basement or applied outside, it does have a very negative effect on our health.

But toxins affect more than just your family — they also affect pets. Three-quarters of dogs tested have chemicals in their urine after lawns were treated with toxins — which increases their chances of getting cancer by about 70%. We must stop using toxins indoors *and* outdoors. Let's take a closer look at the toxins' effects on the yard and the many other toxins present in the basement and garage.

TOXINS PRESENT

Mold

Often found in damp spaces with poor airflow, molds are found indoors in areas such as bathrooms, basements, and garages, and in wet outdoor areas, such as forests, ponds, leaves, and dead trees. Mold spores cannot be seen with the naked eye, and when they land on a wet surface and are combined with some heat, they can grow into the mold that can be seen.

Indoors, mold is found on roofs, in pipes, walls, plant pots, and wet paper or cardboard. It is relatively common in buildings, especially in areas that receive a lot of rainfall or go through flooding. Certain toxic products like paints, insulation, drywall, and carpets can promote mold growth. It can be prevented indoors with the help of bathroom fans, dehumidifiers, and portable fans that keep air flowing through damp areas. And if anything ever springs a leak — pipes, faucets, toilets, fix it right away! Even on a day when you don't need air conditioning or heating, keep the exchange on to keep air moving through the home, as it will help to keep mold from developing.

Another concern for developing mold is condensation. Areas such as bathrooms or low spots in the basements can have persistent condensation if fans are not utilized enough. Condensation builds when warm and cold air collide — bathrooms tend to warm up quickly, and the cold walls can collect moisture (this is also a concern for homes with lead paint, as condensation can cause paint layers to peel).

Most people don't suffer instantly from mold. However, over time, it can cause skin irritations, headaches, rashes, wheezing, and mold-related infections such as sporotrichosis and histoplasmosis. People who suffer from allergies are most likely to suffer from symptoms earlier than those who don't.

Mold can be cleaned naturally with white vinegar and tea tree oil.

Found In:	Alternative/Solution:
Pipes	Monthly run very hot water followed by vinegar through all drains (e.g. kitchen, bathrooms, and laundry room sinks)
Insulation	When renovating, make sure there is a cm or two between the floor and the bottom of the drywall. It will be covered with trim, but it will be enough to keep some airflow going through the insulation and prevent mold.
Roofs and clay tiles	Have them professionally cleaned every two years or sooner if you notice potential mold growth
Home gardens and yards	Keep a spacious layout throughout so that there is plenty of airflow. In the fall, rake all leaves and create a compost pile. Once decomposed, if you wish, you can respread on the ground as a fertilizer.

Carbon Monoxide

How often have you started your car on a cold winter day to warm it up before you drive out into the elements? Unfortunately, when you don't lift the garage door beforehand, the levels of carbon monoxide rise quickly. Since it is odorless and colorless, an unsuspecting person can easily be harmed by it. It can also be caused by small engines such as lawnmowers and snow blowers.

Symptoms of carbon monoxide poisoning include headaches, dizziness, sweating, and difficulty breathing. In extreme cases, it can lead to death.

Lead*

When you move into a house, what's one thing you can almost always count on being left behind in some back corner of the basement or garage? Paint. The old crusty paint cans sit on the shelf just in case some touch-up paint is required. But when the walls are repainted, how often do we reuse the cans? It's time to toss them — and it's probably one of the easiest things you could ever dispose of!

It is always best to avoid working and interacting with lead by enlisting the help of a professional painter. Professional refers to a company certified in removing or covering up lead paint, not a buddy who does painting as a side job on the weekends. Without a professional, you can increase your exposure to it, which can lead to cognitive issues, decreased IQ, behavioral issues, reproductive system damage, increased blood pressure, and anemia.

Found In:	Alternative/Solution:
Paint	Lead-free and VOC-free paint

Asbestos*

Like lead, asbestos is best removed by professionals. You should get it professionally tested if you live in an older home. Asbestos is often found in window caulking and glazing, HVAC duct insulation, plaster, older stove tops, vinyl flooring (tiles and adhesive), artificial embers for gas-fired fireplaces, and textured paint. It is linked to lung cancer, asbestosis, and mesothelioma.

Found In:	Alternative/Solution:
Window caulking and glazing, HVAC duct insulation, plaster, older stove tops, vinyl flooring (tiles and adhesive), artificial embers for gas-fired fireplaces, and textured paint	Live in a home newer than 1980. If the home is older, consider getting it tested and then decide from there what course of action you'll follow.

Radon

Radon has not yet been discussed in this book, so let's dive deep into what it is. Radon is a gas found in 20 to 30% of homes. This natural gas is colorless and odorless, making it dangerous since many people are unaware it is present in the home or air. In the great outdoors, it disperses quickly, but when trapped indoors, it can build up over time. Radon slips inside through cracks in the foundation, walls, fireplaces, and furnaces; outside, it can be found in groundwater, surface water, rocks, and soil.

Radon is a very serious radioactive gas that is linked to lung cancer – the EPA (Environmental Protection Agency) believes that 21,000 people die every year in the USA from radon-related lung cancer. [1]

There are now home radon test kits available. If you live in an area (such as Utah) that is prone to radon poisoning, it is recommended that you periodically get your home tested. If you find high radon levels in your home, the short-term solution is to open windows and get a few fans running. This should dissipate the radon fairly quickly; however, in the long term, you'll need to install a radon reduction ventilation system and seal all cracks in your foundation.

Found In:	Alternative/Solution:
Comes through foundational and wall cracks	Seal all cracks and install a radon reduction ventilation system.

Car Mats

Once, I found myself at a big box store in search of new car mats. As I approached them in the aisle, the undeniable stench coming from them was instantly giving me a headache. I read the label which, plain as day, said, 'May Cause Cancer and Birth Defects or Other Reproductive Harm.' The smell was so incredibly strong that I'm sure it would be true. Needless to say, I did not purchase any mats that day.

Inexpensive car mats often contain VOCs, phthalates, and heavy metals. While driving in a car with the windows down, you can imagine the amount of indoor pollution you are exposed to on your short trips.

Opt for natural or synthetic rubber or TPE mats.

OUTDOORS

The great outdoors thrived for thousands of years without the help of toxins. Today, radon, pesticides, and insecticides fill the soil, and big corporations try to push every nutrient out of the ground in a single crop. To do that, they try to kill anything and everything that may 'harm' the plant – such as biology in the soil and native plants.

Chlorine

The hot summer sun beats down on you as you jump into the pool. You spend several blissful hours playing with friends in the water before heading home for dinner — barbequed burgers and corn salad. It was the perfect summer day. And one that repeated every day for the whole summer.

For many, countless hours are spent at the community pool or spray park, cooling off in the water. A few weeks in, everyone starts to slather themselves with lotions to keep the dry skin to a minimum.

Along with skin irritations, chlorine is also known to negatively impact virtually every system of the body, including low blood pressure, many cancers, asthma, infertility, fibroids, and brain damage. The summers at the pool may have caused more damage to our health than we realized.

A study done in Belgium highlighted the impact of swimming in chlorine. Children who spent a lot of time in pools were eight times more likely to get asthma or to develop allergies. [2]

However, chlorine is found in more than pool water—cleaning products — such as those found in garages and pools. Chlorine byproducts include chloroform. If you don't have a filter on your water at the source where it enters your home, add shower filters to the shower heads to clean the water.

HOW TO LOWER THE IMPACT OF CHLORINE

Spending too much time in chlorine waters can cause 'chlorine itch.' It is a condition where your skin and hair dry out because of constant contact with water. Many kids who spend time at local pools and professional swimmers suffer from this. Adults who spend much time in their hot tubs also suffer from it.

1. Wear a swimmer's cap while swimming in pools. This will prevent the chlorine from stripping the hair of its natural oils and prevent the scalp from peeling (commonly referred to as dandruff).

2. Wear goggles. Ever have red eyes after swimming? You can thank that to the chlorine water. Wearing goggles adds a protective shield to your eyes, which is one of the four ways substances can enter the body.

3. Apply lotion, skin butter, or toxin-free sunscreen. This will create a layer of protection between you and the chlorine.

4. Showering before and after you enter the pool. Pools recommend you wash before entering the pool to help keep the pool clean, but it also adds a level of protection for you as that first contact with water, which helps to moisten the skin. When you enter the water, a slight barrier has already been formed — after all, the skin can only absorb so much water. Then, showering afterward will help wash off excess chlorine before the skin absorbs it.

5. Diving suits. The more skin you cover up that doesn't have access to water, the safer your skin will be. Diving suits tend to cover up the body and protect it from the elements — cold and chlorine.

Found In:	Alternative/Solution:
Swimming pools	Saltwater pools, ocean or lake water

Whether you have a backyard pool or attend a local community pool, consider the option of saltwater pools. They are much safer than chlorine (although they can still dry out the skin and hair) and often come with the same price tag as chlorine pools. You can also add in oxidation systems, which reduce the need for products in the water anywhere from 30% to 70%. Another option is to avoid pools and set up a backyard sprinkler or slip-and-slide using a garden hose with a filtration system.

PESTICIDES & INSECTICIDES

"A Who's Who of pesticides is therefore of concern to us all. If we are going to live so intimately with these chemicals, eating and drinking them, taking them into the very marrow of our bones - we had better know something about their nature and their power."

— RACHEL CARSON, SILENT SPRING

DETOX: BASEMENT, GARAGE, & OUTDOORS

The use of pesticides and insecticides has become a common practice in both agriculture and pest control. While these chemicals effectively control pests and increase crop yields, they come with substantial health risks associated with their use. Pesticides and insecticides contain harmful chemicals that can have detrimental effects on our health when we are exposed to them. This section will explore how these substances can be toxic to our health and the importance of minimizing our exposure to them.

'Pesticide' and 'insecticide' are both generic terms and can be used to describe the purpose of a substance. A pesticide is a compound used to kill pests and insects that may harm plants – unfortunately, it kills most biology in the ground. An insecticide is a type of pesticide that focuses on killing insects. Because it can be made up of different substances, the side effects of pesticides and insecticides vary. They can enter the body through the skin, inhalation, oral, and eyes. Short-term side effects are headaches, abdominal pain (vomiting, diarrhea, cramps), fatigue, blindness, dizziness, and weakness. Long-term and more severe symptoms include congenital disabilities, tumors, blood and nerve disorders, cancer, and endocrine disruptors.

Warning Labels

Pesticides, insecticides, and herbicides come with different warning labels. Some of these include:

- Poison – highly toxic and contains a skull and crossbones symbol
- Danger – very toxic and contains skull and crossbones symbols (similar to poison and sometimes used interchangeably)

- Warning – moderately toxic but still potentially fatal
- Caution – contains lower doses but still could be deadly

Pesticides and herbicides spread beyond the substances you spray on your lawn and garden. Buying non-organic foods can also introduce them to your system, and they are not easy to detox. Home gardens can be much safer without commercially produced pesticides and herbicides. Much of certain types of food grown today is genetically modified, and as Jim Marrs, who wrote *Population Control: How Corporate Owners Are Killing Us*, highlighted, they are only getting more potent: "Over 80 percent of all GMOs grown worldwide are engineered for herbicide tolerance. As a result, the use of toxic herbicides like Roundup has increased fifteen times since GMOs were introduced. GMO crops are also responsible for the emergence of 'superweeds' and 'superbugs': which can only be killed with ever more toxic poisons."

Found In:	Alternative/Solution:
Pesticides, herbicides, and insecticides	Plant-based compost, thyme oil, clove oil, peppermint oil
Non-Organic Foods	Organic and non-GMO crops.

TOXIC PLANTS

One area that often goes unnoticed is the presence of toxic plants that can pose a threat to both pets and ourselves. Most plants are beautiful and a pleasure to be around. Adults typically don't have any issues with toxic plans, but pets and children sometimes do, given their tendency to chew on things. Avoid having the following plants in your yard if you have pets or young children. And avoid eating any plants until you 100%

confirm what it is and that they are edible. Side effects of eating toxic plants can lead to diarrhea, vomiting, weakness, and lethargy.

Having a generic understanding that some plants can be toxic, when we look into each plant, we can recall the information better and protect our pets and ourselves — it's one more way to keep the members of your home safe. With this knowledge, we can enjoy our surroundings without worrying about potential hazards that could harm those we care about.

This section will explore various types of toxic plants for both pets and humans. We will delve into their specific dangers and provide valuable insights on how to prevent any unfortunate incidents from occurring.

Aloe Vera — Toxic for pets but not humans, aloe vera contains polysaccharides and phenolic chemicals, which can cause them to vomit, cramp, and have diarrhea. In severe cases, it can cause kidney failure.

Amaryllis – The amaryllis plant contains a toxin called lycorine, a crystalline alkaloid that can be deadly if consumed in larger quantities. Lycorine causes drooling and severe stomach pain, which produces flu-like symptoms.

Autumn crocus – Also known as wild saffron, autumn crocuses are purple flowers that contain a toxin called alkaloid colchicine, which can be fatal.

Azalea – Azaleas contain grayanotoxins; even low quantities can cause severe stomach pain.

Castor bean — A toxin without an antidote, ricin, is a natural toxin found in castor beans. If a pet or child consumes this plant, seek immediate health care attention.

Chrysanthemum — Often found in fresh flower bouquets, chrysanthemums contain sesquiterpene lactones and pyrethrins, two ingredients found in insecticides.

Cyclamen — Cyclamens have terpenoid saponins and can cause severe stomach pains.

Daffodil — One of the first spring flowers, daffodils contain the toxin called lycorine — the same toxin as the Amaryllis.

Dieffenbachia — more than an outdoor plant, today, the dieffenbachia is a prevalent indoor plant. Symptoms include swelling of the tongue and blisters in the mouth. It can also cause abdominal pains.

English ivy — One of the less toxic plants on this list; however, it abounds everywhere in humid areas, making it more likely that pets will come into contact with it. It contains saponins, which can cause abdominal pain and vomiting and, in extreme cases, coma and death.

Hyacinth - Like many of the bulb perennials on this list, the hyacinth contains lactones and alkaloids in large quantities in the bulb. Even when humans handle the bulbs, they should wear gloves to protect themselves from the toxins.

Hydrangea - Hydrangeas contain cyanide, a very toxic substance. Consuming small doses can lead to dizziness, difficulty breathing, and fainting. In severe cases, it can cause death.

Jade plant - The jade plant is unique because it is one of the few plants we know is toxic, but we don't know why. Its symp-

DETOX: BASEMENT, GARAGE, & OUTDOORS

toms are mysterious: irregular heartbeat, vomiting, and diarrhea. It can be poisonous to the touch, so always wear gloves while handling them, and if you accidentally touch any part of the plant, wash your hands thoroughly with water and soap.

Lily and Peace Lilies – These plants contain calcium oxalates, which can impact the appetite and cause dehydration, vomiting, and diarrhea. In extremely rare and severe cases, it can cause liver failure.

Nerium oleander – The poisonous pink beauty, which contains oleandrin, nerin, digitoxigenin, olinerin, and rosagenin, none of which should be digested. Just a single leaf is toxic enough to kill an adult. Let's sum it up by saying, stay away.

Philodendron – Another common houseplant, philodendrons contain calcium oxalate, like lilies. The symptoms are the same.

Poinsettia – The ever-popular Christmas flower is slightly toxic and shouldn't be mixed with your salad greens. However, besides vomiting and possible diarrhea, the poinsettia is one of the safer toxic plants.

Sago palm – The sago palm is very dangerous for pets — as in death, as little as fifteen minutes of consumption. Immediate symptoms include vomiting and diarrhea, but it can cause quick liver failure when consumed in high doses.

Spider Plant – While not very toxic and unlikely to cause death, the spider plant is a hallucinogenic. So, while a pet might act a little crazy because they see or hear things that aren't there, for the most part, they will be fine once it works through their system.

Tulip – the tulip contains lactones and alkaloids in large quantities in the bulb, just like the hyacinth and the daffodil.

Widow's-thrill – This plant contains bufadienolides, which affect the cardiovascular system. If left untreated, it can lead to cardiac arrest and death. Early symptoms of bufadienolide poisoning include feeling cold, vomiting, and diarrhea.

Yew - The yew plant contains several toxins that can cause serious harm. Interestingly enough, though, it is mostly only poisonous in the winter.

Poisons and toxins, whether natural or found in herbicides, pesticides, and insecticides, impact your health, and by removing them from your life, your health can only improve.

Toxins and sources of toxins can be found in the basement and the outdoor areas of a house, such as the yard, pool, and car. We have now gone through every area of the home, and you have the knowledge to make informed decisions for you and your family.

FIVE THINGS YOU CAN DO TODAY:

❖ Check the labels of everything you have in the garage. While there are no clean alternatives for some things, such as car oil or antifreeze, products you apply to your yard and garden have green substitutes.
❖ Stop using chlorine pools and hot tubs and opt for salt water instead. If chlorine pools are necessary, always shower before and after and apply a non-toxic lotion or sunblock to prevent chlorine from breaking the skin barrier.

DETOX: BASEMENT, GARAGE, & OUTDOORS

❖ Get rid of all herbicides, pesticides, and insecticides; they can harm you, your family, pets, food, and much more.

❖ Avoid having poisonous plants in your home or gardens if you have children and pets. Their damage can range from minimal to severe.

❖ Familiarize yourself with toxin symbols to know what kind of danger each level presents.

PART III

TAKING CONTROL

8

MAKING CHANGES

After analyzing the toxins in each room of your home, you are now very much aware of the personal and environmental health risks posed by manufactured products. And I hope this has translated into some positive changes.

69% of all global consumers admit to being advocates for zero-waste. In fact, the movement for zero-waste packaging is expected to grow by 13.2% from 2021 to 2026.

According to a marketing report by McKinsey, "Gen Z" shoppers (or people born between 1996 and 2010) are more likely to spend their money on brands that appear to be ethical.[1] Another similar report states that 66% of consumers are content to spend more on products that come from sustainable brands. That said, companies have a financial incentive to be – or at least appear to be – socially conscious.

As a result of consumers desiring to be more green, many companies are now starting to use it as a marketing tactic, or at the very least guilt tripping consumers into purchasing their products by making them feel that they are responsible for all the terrible toxins that have been released into the environment which ironically is mostly the businesses fault.

Greenwashing has become a marketing sensation since the early 2000s despite the term first being used in 1986 by an environmentalist. It refers to marketing tactics that promote a product's efficiency and lower environmental impacts — however, these statements are false or very misleading. Sometimes, greenwashing can be subtle, but other times, it is blatantly obvious. For example, packaging that includes green foliage can give the impression that a company is nature-based, thereby leaving the consumer with the impression that the product is safe for themselves and the environment. However, a not-so-obvious tactic would be to ask hotel or pool guests to reuse their towels to protect the environment when, in reality, it is a money-saving endeavor for the facilities to do less laundry and put a few extra dollars in their pockets. A better alternative would be replacing all the shower heads, taps, and toilets with water-efficient ones, but that would cost the hotels and pools millions of dollars rather than the cost of a piece of paper with a notice that essentially instructs the customer to save the facilities money.

MARKETING LANGUAGE

 "Advertising: the science of arresting the human intelligence long enough to get money from it."

— STEPHEN LEACOCK

Knowing the language that marketing teams use to promote their 'green-ness' is critical to weed out the companies that are actually green and those that are not. The first point of reference should always be reading the product labels, as the empty terminology on the packaging should always be a caution sign to be alert. Popular terms and phrases include:

- Eco-friendly
- Produced sustainably
- X% greener than leading brands
- Working to be more sustainable
- Greening
- X% less emissions
- Be clean, go green
- Green
- Clean
- Earth
- Recycle
- Good for the planet/environment
- Less is more
- Green targets
- Manufactured sustainably
- Made from recycled materials
- Made from renewable sources

One common theme among these terms is that they are vague and often have nothing to do with the product itself or have no facts to back up their claims. It pays to pretend to be green, as most people are willing to pay a few extra cents or dollars if a product is 'green.'

Images to be cautious of:

- Trees, leaves, flowers
- Foliage
- Tractors, farms
- Planet
- Green (color)

Today, organizations adopt all sorts of 'greener' tactics, from green energy to tree planting schemes. While green energy sounds great, in reality, some methods use excessive amounts of oil to run, are not compostable, and can use lithium. This very toxic chemical can cause significant pollution to bodies of water. Both are a danger to animals.

In addition, large corporations frequently use factories and sweatshops to develop and produce their products, and clothing companies specializing in fast fashion are especially prone to this. Avoiding large retailers and corporations (who don't become wealthy by saving the environment and your health) is just one way to avoid toxins.

Some companies desire to move away from oil and gas since many assume this is more dangerous for the environment than batteries. However, batteries contain a variety of toxins that are mined throughout the world and then shipped to factories to be assembled. Lithium is just one of the minerals mined, a type of mining done deep in the earth's crust. In 2016, 211.3 million metric tons of carbon emissions were the result of lithium mining[2], and with the continued demand for technologies, that number only goes up. This is just one toxin released into the atmosphere for a simple thing such as batteries. There are thousands of toxins that also need to be mined, combined, and mixed to create the goods and services we use on a daily basis. This is just one of the many reasons why we need to be aware of what goes on 'behind the scenes' of organizations who promote their 'green-ness' or try to guilt-trip their customers into buying green, when, in reality, the customers are only paying more because of a marketing tactic.

Greenwashing is all around us, but there are ways to determine if a company is being honest rather than being vague to ensure that customers will buy their products. Over the years, here is how I have learned when to assume companies are telling the truth and when they are being honest.

Clear language: When a package says 'Made with 97% natural ingredients' rather than 'Made with organic ingredients,' it uses clear language. Clear language tells you exactly what is inside rather than leads you to make assumptions about it that are often false when investigated.

Comparison checks: If a product is from a big-name corporation, most likely, there are competitors who have similar products. For example, when you walk down the laundry detergent aisle at the grocery store, you'll notice three to four big brands, all with similar products. If Company X has a 'natural' detergent for $15, but Company Y has a similar one for $20, the price discrepancy is probably related to the ingredients used and their manufacturing practices. Therefore, while both may be 'natural,' it is vital to check the ingredients to see which one is actually more 'natural.'

Data: If the packaging contains statistics such as 'America's leading brand' or '94% of consumers prefer X over Y', then look for website links that verify the stat. Another critical factor is to look for a website address and a proper mailing address on the package.

Images: Ask yourself, if this was in a black box with the name and a list of the ingredients in clear English, would it still be enticing based on the purpose and ingredients of a product? If not, then the images on the packaging are likely influencing your decision.

TECHNOLOGY VS TOXINS

Most of society has chosen to live with technology (myself included) as it makes our lives easier and more enjoyable. Laptops, cell phones, tablets, earbuds, and televisions are very much ingrained in our lifestyles. We know how these can affect our attention span and how blue light affects our circadian rhythm. Since we have decided to use technology, we might as well use what we choose to benefit us by helping us live in a cleaner, more toxin-free environment.

Today, there are dozens of resources dedicated solely to living toxin-free. This would include blogs, YouTube channels, and apps. The first two vary significantly in reliability, but let's talk about some apps that help us to quickly identify how safe ingredients are.

- ❖ **Think Dirty App** – Love makeup? Love the idea of toxin-free makeup? This app allows you to scan the barcodes of makeup and gives you a toxicity level and a list of the ingredients and toxins found in them!
- ❖ **CosDNA** – if you like spreadsheets, this is your app!

Packed with data, this app highlights all the details on toxins in beauty products.

❖ **Detox Me** – an app that gives tips and tricks to detoxing your home while allowing you to track your progress.

❖ **CosmEthics** – Another makeup app, this one tracks not only toxins but also possible allergies.

❖ **Yuka** – the app that tracks toxins found in the aisles of the grocery store and gives them a rank of poor, bad, good, and excellent — and presents you with better alternatives.

❖ **Clearya** – an excellent app for those who like to shop online at major retailers such as Amazon and Target and sends notifications if a product contains toxic ingredients.

❖ **EWG Healthy Living** – created by the Environmental Working Group, this app tracks the toxins in major household products. It's as simple as scanning a barcode and getting a rating (on a scale of one to ten) of how good the product is. EWG's website was one of the first I encountered on my toxin-free journey. It covers everything from cosmetics and cleaners to food and water. To this day, it is still my favorite.

❖ **INCIDecoder** – One toxin can have multiple names, and the INCIDecoder helps you sort out exactly what is in products.

One of the first apps I downloaded was the Yuka app, and for fun, I began by going through my fridge and pantry, scanning each item, and reading the rating it got. A couple of items that I thought were relatively healthy only received a 15-20 point range (out of the possible 100)! It stunned me that although I thought I ate very healthily, there was something even I had fallen for in terms of marketing schemes. My favorite 'healthy' salad dressing scored lower than my favorite 'junk' food! It was an eye-opening experience highlighting that I should always look at the ingredients and not just the marketing. Every app has its pros and cons, and this one, while it is not perfect, is very beneficial.

NATURAL LIVING

> "Many 'pathogens' (both chemical and behavioral) can influence how you turn out; these include substance abuse by a mother during pregnancy, maternal stress, and low birth weight. As a child grows, neglect, physical abuse, and head injury can cause problems in mental development. Once the child is grown, substance abuse and exposure to a variety of toxins can damage the brain, modifying intelligence, aggression, and decision-making abilities. The major public health movement to remove lead-based paint grew out of an understanding that even low levels of lead can cause brain damage that makes children less intelligent and, in some cases, more impulsive and aggressive."
>
> — DAVID EAGLEMAN.[3]

Natural living is a concept that embraces living in an environment free from chemicals and toxins while also being organic and sustainable. In essence, we aim not to leave a footprint behind us that will cause harm to future generations. In the best-case scenario, we are continually improving or bettering our environment and are setting those future generations up for successes greater than our own. We want to live lives that run in sync with nature and not against it. For example, we eat fruit, not an artificial fruit snack, or buy products in glass jars, not plastic, whenever possible.

We live in a world of abundance, and because of this, it is easy to adopt a maximalist mentality. While minimalism may be an extreme, when we focus on living naturally, we aim to buy what we use and leave what we don't. We don't shop just for the sake of shopping and focus on purchasing items that we can continually reuse, have a long shelf life, or can be purchased secondhand in still very good condition. One of the largest wastes today is food and plastics — every year, millions of tons of food is thrown out, and only 9% of plastic is recycled. Ask yourself, what can I do to reduce food waste? How can I reduce my product consumption? We all have weaknesses and things we love to buy. Personally, I loved buying all the kitchen gadgets one can dream of. Different peels, organizers, spatulas, shredders, if I could get it in quantities, I did. Even if the gadget I bought wasn't the best, I loved adding it to the collection. Over my years of aiming to live more naturally, I had to withhold myself from buying new gadgets until I wore out the 30-plus useless gadgets I seldom use — let's say it was several years' worth of supplies! In time, I have decided quality is much better than quantity!

Sometimes, things can seem to be sacrifices, but today, I know that the materials I purchase are *needed* and will be *used* rather than sitting in storage for years to come with the hope that one day I can use them before it goes out of style. My gadget addiction may be a bit of a stretch, but I hope it drives home the point that we all have areas to cut back on! What do you need to cut back on?

Natural Living Principles

There are many different interpretations and principles for living naturally, but the following has become a foundational part of my life over the years. While not set in stone, they are the overarching guiding principles of natural living that I try to adhere to — and of course, it's all with the aim of being natural, toxin-free, and sustainable.

1. Focus on what is real. Whether food, furniture, or home goods, I always aim to buy the real thing, not imitation or knock-off goods. Avoid fast food, fast fashion, and hot trends. What we buy is what we use or will last us for decades to come.

2. Focus on what is healthy. Living a toxin-free life that focuses on being healthy is a lifelong goal, and natural health is always preferred over synthetic ways. This means that I focus on natural household cleaners and organic and non-GMO foods but also avoid excess screen time, go to bed on time, exercise regularly, and get outdoor time.

3. Focus on what is mindful. My family and I have what we need and a few extra items, but we don't live extravagantly or allow ourselves to become hoarders. If we don't need it, we don't buy it; if we no longer need it, we give it away.

4. Focus on what is local. Locally grown products are not on most people's list of natural living; however, when focusing on living toxin-free, we must realize the price of distance. A carton

MAKING CHANGES

of blueberries that travels 1,500 miles has a much larger carbon footprint than the one from the farmer down the road or at the farmer's market. Those 1,500-mile blueberries also need toxins to be preserved or picked before they are ripe and then sprayed to ripen.

Choosing to live naturally is freeing. It brings peace of mind and restores the body. For thousands of years, the human race lived this way, and arguably, it's only been since the '90s and the rise of the Internet and on-demand services and year-round availability that we have, by and large, forgotten how to live this way.

Detoxing our homes is much more than just removing the chemical toxins. It's a lifestyle that focuses on being whole and allowing our bodies to function as they should. There are natural alternatives that can be used rather than chemical or synthetic ones. You can make products rather than purchase them. You can live with the seasons, having quiet periods and busy times.

You can protect your body and the earth from further harm. You can change the future.

Natural living needs to be your way forward. It has short- and long-term benefits, but the primary reason should be for your physical and mental health. Many people notice that they lose weight, become in better shape, and have clearer skin while having their brain fog disappear (I myself am a testament to that!). It will improve your outlook on life, and you will be stronger mentally.

As you become reconnected with who you are and with nature, you will begin to see a simpler and less stressful way of life. But, perhaps one of the greatest blessings is the contentment it brings.

DIY NATURAL LIVING

There are many ways you can DIY yourself into natural living. As we near the end of this book, I want to take a few moments to outline practical ways you can adopt natural living practices today. Void from this list are recipes for cleaners — those you will find in the bonus chapter focusing on cleaner and greener household cleaners and personal care items!

1. Reduce and reuse. It's time to say goodbye to disposable items and replace them with lasting alternatives. From plastic wraps to diapers and feminine products, there are numerous ways you can start reducing your waste today.

2. Buy bulk goods. Sometimes, organic, toxin-free goods can be more costly than the alternative. Therefore, as your budget allows, purchase bulk items to help you save money.

3. Eat real food. As I mentioned earlier, eating real food is always better than the alternative. This would be eating eggs rather than eggs from a carton, raw honey rather than fructose, and an orange rather than bottled orange juice.

4. Cooking and baking from scratch. When you make food from scratch, you know exactly what goes into the meal. From the farm-fresh carrots and potatoes to the local beef tossed with fresh herbs and spices, meals can easily be toxin-free. Over the years, I have established a handful of favorite recipes and can make them with minimal effort at the end of a long day. Come up with a few family favorites and ensure you always have those ingredients on hand; toxin-free cooking will become second nature.

5. Start a green community. Teaching others about the dangers of toxins is a great way to create a lasting change. Consider starting a local group, either in person or online, such as a WhatsApp or FaceBook group, to encourage each other or to swap ideas. If you are comfortable, you could also ask people if you could speak to them (and their friends!) about toxin-free living for an hour. The most successful people are those who create a tribe of like-minded people around themselves.

When I decided to get healthy, this is precisely what I did. I knew that I would need a support group for long-term success, and since I couldn't find one that fit my needs, I created one. It started off small — just a few friends — who came over for a 'Healthy Party'. Everyone brought a healthy food item, and being eco-friendly was strongly encouraged. What started out as a small group of seven eventually grew to more than thirty!

6. Get moving. Exercise keeps your body and mind healthy by improving cardiovascular strength, stretching muscles, and circulating blood. It releases endorphins that will enhance your mental outlook while also helping you sleep better.

Five Things You Can Do Today:

- ❖ Download one of the apps previously mentioned and test it out on products in your fridge, pantry, or bathroom.
- ❖ Focus on using up products in your home rather than shopping for new products (unless they are toxic and you have the means to change them right away).

- Research local farmers and farmer markets – make a plan to visit them!
- Make a WhatsApp group with friends who you feel are like-minded and start sharing your knowledge and ideas.
- Come up with one recipe every week for four weeks that you fine-tune to make it a quick-and-easy meal.

CONCLUSION

Your home is your safe oasis and should be free from toxins. From laundry detergents to shampoo to non-stick pans, we have allowed toxins to enter our home, which slowly chip away at our good health. However, as you now know, toxins are detrimental to our health, and we do not need them in our homes. There are millions of healthier alternatives than toxic products.

Now that you know the challenge of finding and eliminating household toxins, you know what tools, techniques, and knowledge you need to be up to the task. We have gone from room to room — kitchen, living room, bathrooms, bedrooms — highlighting the common toxins found in each of them, and also provided alternatives and solutions for mitigating them from the room.

Over the last century, thousands of toxins and chemical compounds have been created and are now found in thousands of household items. With consumerism rising and the desire for low prices, many people and organizations substitute quality (and safety) for quality parts and ingredients with toxin and chemical alternatives. It's time to say "No more" to this way of living and return to quality living. And, now that you know the options available, you can start making small but positive — and effective! — changes to minimize your family's exposure to household toxins.

This book has been packed with information about toxins found in your home. If you found this book helpful, please leave a review about your experience with it where you purchased it. This will help others become aware of the book and change to a toxin-free lifestyle as well. Please also recommend it to friends and family!

As you transition from toxins to toxin-free, do not overwhelm yourself by doing it all in one day. Transition as cleaning products and self-care items run out, and replace them with non-toxic options (unless your budget allows for a quicker switch). Take it all one day and one product at a time. When in doubt, you can refer back to this book for guidance.

Remember to discuss the changes and the need for a toxin-free home with everyone in the home so the toxins don't get accidentally brought back into it. After the initial conversation, rather than continually lecturing (which probably won't be effective), adding one-line comments such as 'Grab the green bottle, that one is chemical free' will help to reinforce the idea over time. The way forward is in a home that is toxin-free. If you haven't started detoxing it yet, start today!

The final appendix is a quick list of where you can start. Your life has begun to change, and I hope you can already see a bigger, brighter future.

CONCLUSION

Join my email list for updates on non-toxic living, DIY recipe ideas, product recommendations, sustainable living tips, gut health information, and more.

www.wellnessreclaimed.com/secrets

I look forward to meeting you once again in the next book in this series!

BONUS CHAPTER: DIY RECIPES

MAKING AND TAKING CARE OF YOUR COSMETICS

Making homemade cosmetics is not complicated, but it does have a learning curve. Understanding these basic concepts will make it much more manageable. You'll find that you can make once and have enough products to last months at a time.

When creating homemade recipes, always aim to use the best possible ingredients. The higher the quality of these ingredients — such as organic and non-GMO — the higher the quality of the end product. Using non-organic ingredients can result in the products not being completely toxin-free.

Preservative-Free

Most preservatives are not natural, and the ones that are natural are not that easy to use. If you would like to add a preservative to your cosmetics, you will have to research it independently. Preservatives must be added to a product once water is added, or else it must be kept in the fridge and consumed within a few days. Items that are not water-based do not require a preservative, and with proper care, can last up to 6 months or more.

Extending Shelf Life Naturally

Always use clean hands when using your finished products or a spoon to scoop them out to avoid contamination. Also, please do not leave the cosmetic in a hot area or where the temperature may change dramatically, as this could cause it to go bad. Always store cosmetics in dark jars or containers and away from direct sunlight. That being said, I've had whipped body butter for six-plus months, with my family using them as well, and have not had any problems.

Double Boiler

Many cosmetics, such as lotion bars, whipped body butter, lip balms, etc., require the raw ingredients to be warmed up and melted. To do this, you need to make a double boiler. A double boiler is simply a glass or stainless steel bowl in a pan/pot of water on the stove. The heated water warms up the ingredients. This prevents the ingredients (butter/oils/waxes) from getting too much heat and burning.

As with anything in the kitchen, do not leave your ingredients on the stove unattended. If heated too high, certain oils can catch on fire. Also, certain kinds of butter, such as shea, can become grainy if heated excessively or at a high temperature.

Clean up

Cleaning up after using butters and oils can be challenging if you don't know where to start. First, start by using a spatula and getting as much of your warm butter and oil off as possible. If the ingredients have cooled and hardened, reheat them for easy removal. Then, wipe the bowl and spoons off with a paper towel. Wash dishes with hot, soapy water and stick them in the dishwasher, if needed.

Quantities

You'll find that many of my recipes do not use a specific amount but rather a percentage or fraction. The reasoning behind this is that you can decide how much you want to make. You may want to fill a specific container or make multiple containers (homemade cosmetics make great gifts!) Just make it easy for yourself and assign a tablespoon or some other standard measuring cup or spoon to represent either a certain percentage, like 10%, or a fraction, like a ⅓.

*Notes:

- Common semi-soft butters are shea and mango.
- Common hard butter is cocoa butter.
- Common soft butters are olive, hemp, and avocado.
- Carrier oils are used to moisturize your skin and dilute essential oils. Examples of carrier oils are sweet almond oil, camellia seed oil, jojoba oil, coconut oil, avocado oil, argan oil, and hemp seed oil.

*I always say, keep things simple. Use what you may already have in the kitchen (avocado, coconut, or olive oil). If you would like to experiment more, feel free to get other oils that have different properties and are suitable for different skin types.

*Some essential oils should not be put on the skin, such as many citrus essential oils. Check warnings and usage of essential oils before adding them to your cosmetics.

HOMEMADE COSMETIC RECIPES

Basic Lotion Bar

Ingredients:

- 1/3 beeswax*
- 1/3 cocoa butter
- 1/3 camellia seed oil, olive oil, apricot kernel oil, sweet almond, jojoba, coconut oil, or other carrier oil
- Essential oils (optional)
- Vitamin E (optional)

* Refer to instructions regarding quantities, carrier oils, and essential oils on the previous page.

Directions:

1. Add beeswax and butter together in a double boiler on medium heat.
2. When melted, add the carrier oil and stir until thoroughly mixed and dissolved.
3. Remove from heat.
4. Add essential oil (one teaspoon to a 9 oz batch) and Vitamin E when the mixture cools slightly.
5. Pour into molds and let harden on the counter or refrigerator.
6. Remove from molds when completely set, then store away from light and heat.
7. To use, rub onto skin. Your skin's warmth will soften the bar and moisturize you.

Whipped Body Butter

Ingredients:

- 2/3 shea butter (or a combination of preferred semi-soft or soft butters)
- 1/3 preferred carrier oil(s)
- Essential oils (optional)
- Vitamin E (optional)

Directions:

1. Melt butter in a double boiler.
2. When melted, add the carrier oil and stir until completely combined.
3. Remove from heat and cool slightly before adding essential oils and vitamin E. Mix together.
4. Allow the mixture to harden, and then repeat whipping with an electric mixer until the desired consistency is achieved.
5. Transfer to your container.

* If using a whisk, place the bowl in the refrigerator for 10 minutes, remove and beat by hand. Repeat mixing and refrigerating for half an hour. To keep the butter from hardening, beat the mixture 2-3 times for the next two days. Transfer into your container.

* In warmer months, you may choose to use more butters and less carrier oils, 4/5 Butters and 1/5 oils. Or you may choose to make it without any oils at all.

* **Alternate directions:** Place all ingredients in a mixing bowl and do not heat. Beat with an electric mixer or whisk until fully combined and the desired consistency is reached.

Hand and Body Scrub Option #1 (Most Popular)

Ingredients:

- Olive oil 15%
- Coconut oil 15%
- Camellia seed oil 15%
- Fractionated coconut oil 15% (or regular coconut oil)
- Cocoa butter 15%
- Shea butter/mango butter 15%
- Olive butter/avocado butter 5 %
- Hemp seed butter 5%
- Essential oils
- Sugar

Directions:

1. In a double boiler, melt butter completely, then add carrier oils. When completely melted, remove from heat and stir.
2. Allow to cool to room temperature, and then add essential oils.
3. Add in enough white sugar until the desired consistency is reached.
4. Take a scoop of scrub on dry hands and rub gently all over. Wash with warm water. Enjoy the soft, moisturized skin!

BONUS CHAPTER: DIY RECIPES

* Feel free to experiment with different carrier oils or butters.

Hand and Body Scrub Option #2

Ingredients:

- 1/2 cup shea butter or a combination of semi-soft and soft butters
- 1/3 cup camellia seed oil/olive oil/coconut oil or other carrier oil
- Essential oil
- White sugar

Directions:

1. In a mixing bowl, blend shea butter (or other butters) with a mixer until creamy and no lumps remain.
2. Add in carrier oil and essential oil and beat again.
3. By hand, mix in sugar until the desired consistency is reached.

Lip Balm

Ingredients:

- 1/5 beeswax
- 2/5 cocoa butter/shea butter/other butter
- 2/5 coconut oil/camellia seed oil/castor oil/olive oil
- Essential oils (optional)

Directions:

1. Melt beeswax and butters in a double boiler.
2. When melted, add carrier oils and mix until well blended.
3. Remove from heat and allow the mixture to cool slightly.
4. Add essential oil.
5. Pour into lip balm tubes or other containers and allow to cool.

* Add more cocoa butter and beeswax for a less emollient and harder lip balm.

* A lip balm tube is usually about 0.17oz

Lip Scrub

Ingredients:

- 2/3 brown sugar
- 1/6 raw cane sugar
- 1/6 turbinado sugar
- Castor oil

Directions:

1. Combine sugars and slowly add in castor oil. Add in just enough oil so the sugar does not easily fall off the spoon.
2. To use, gently rub a small amount of scrub on your lips. Rinse with water.

Facial Cleanser

Ingredients:

- 1/4 cup glycerine
- 1/8 cup honey
- 1 1/2 teaspoon liquid castile soap
- Essential oils (optional)

Directions: Combine all ingredients and mix until well blended.

Deodorant

Ingredients

- 3 Tablespoons coconut oil
- 2 Tablespoons shea butter
- 2 Tablespoons beeswax
- 3 Tablespoons baking soda
- Tablespoon arrowroot powder
- 20 drops Essential oils
- Shelf-stable probiotic powder from 2 pills (optional)
- Powder from 1 capsule of activated charcoal (optional)

Directions:

1. Heat coconut oil, shea butter, and beeswax until melted in a double boiler on medium-low.
2. Remove from heat and add in baking soda, arrowroot powder, probiotic powder, activated charcoal powder, and essential oils.

3. Mix until well combined.
4. Pour the mixture into a container or an old deodorant tube. Allow to cool on the counter or refrigerator.

Emulsion-Free lotion

Ingredients:

- 3 Tablespoons camellia oil or jojoba oil
- 8 drops of essential oil
- Distilled water

Directions:

1. Add Camellia oil and essential oils to a squeeze bottle and shake.
2. Add distilled water to another bottle.
3. Drop five drops of oil mixture on a clean palm and five drops of distilled water and mix with a finger.
4. Apply to face.
5. Adjust the oil-to-water ratio to suit your skin type.

Solid Perfume

Ingredients:

- 1 Tablespoon beeswax
- 1 Tablespoon apricot kernel/jojoba oil
- 8-15 drops essential oil

Directions:

1. Melt beeswax in a double boiler, and then add oil.
2. When thoroughly melted and combined, remove from heat.
3. Allow to cool slightly, and add essential oils.
4. Pour into a container and allow to solidify.

Zit Zapper

Ingredients:

- 1/4 teaspoon apple cider vinegar
- 1 drop of tea tree oil

Directions: Combine ingredients and dab onto the pimple with a cotton ball.

Coconut Toothpaste

Ingredients:

- 3 Tablespoons coconut oil
- 2 Tablespoons baking soda
- 1 Tablespoon arrowroot starch
- 2 Tablespoon xylitol
- 20 drops peppermint/spearmint essential oil
- 1 tablespoon calcium carbonate (optional)

Directions: In a bowl, combine all ingredients until well-mixed. Apply on to toothbrush with a dry applicator and brush as usual.

Foaming Hand Soap

Ingredients:

- 3/10 liquid castile soap
- 7/10 water
- 15-20 drops essential oils (optional)
- Foaming pump soap bottle

Directions: In a foaming soap bottle, add in water, then liquid soap, and finally essential oils. Give it a shake, and it's ready to use!

Hand Sanitizer

Ingredients:

- 3/4 cup isopropyl alcohol (99% strength)
- 10ml hydrogen peroxide
- 50ml distilled water
- 5ml vegetable glycerine
- essential oils (optional)

Directions:

1. Mix all ingredients together, add essential oils if you wish, around 40 drops or less if it reaches the scent potency you like.
2. Mix well.
3. Pour into clean spray bottles.
4. Shake before use. Spray onto your hands whenever you need and rub well.

BONUS CHAPTER: DIY RECIPES

*Do not let children use unsupervised, and ensure hands have dried before eating anything.

DIY CLEANING RECIPES

The following recipes can be used as replacements for many industrial and chemical cleaners. The recipes can easily be doubled or tripled, and if storing them for longer than two months, I recommend that recipes with essential oils be stored in dark glass bottles. All cleaners should be stored in a cool area and out of direct sunlight, and it is recommended they be replaced every six to eight months. When using cleaners, spray or wipe the areas with cleaner and let them sit on the surface for at least fifteen seconds before wiping, as this will give the cleaner a few seconds to work at the dirt and lift it from the surface before you try wiping it.

Notes:

- For recipes with vinegar, do not use them on natural stone, as the acid can eat away at the stone over time.
- Always try to use glass bowls so that the ingredients used in the recipes don't leach into the plastic. Use stainless steel measuring cups and stirring utensils for the same reason.

Tub and Sink Cleaner

Ingredients

- 1 cup white vinegar
- 1/4 cup lemon juice

- 1 tablespoon castile soap
- 10 drops of eucalyptus essential oil
- 5 drops of tea tree essential oil

Instructions

1. In a glass bowl, combine all the ingredients and stir well.
2. Add to a dark spray bottle and apply to tubs and sinks as needed.

Scented All-Purpose Cleaner

Ingredients

- 1 cup white vinegar
- 1 cup water
- 1 Tablespoon lemon juice
- 1 teaspoon castile soap
- 10 drops of rosemary essential oil

Instructions

1. In a glass bowl, combine all the ingredients and stir well.
2. Add to a glass jar or spray bottle and shake it before letting it rest for three to four days to combine the ingredients thoroughly.

Suitable for:

- All-purpose cleaning (surface areas, stove tops, floors, etc.)
- Removing water stains

- Stainless steel
- Spot cleaning walls
- Areas with unpleasant smells (trash cans, wet clothes)

DIY Glass Cleaner

Ingredients

- 1 cup filtered water
- 1/4 cup white vinegar
- 1/4 cup rubbing alcohol
- 5 to 10 drops of eucalyptus essential oil

Instructions

1. Add all of the ingredients to a spray bottle and shake to combine all ingredients..
2. If using the mixture to clean windows with a rag, wear gloves so it doesn't dry out your hands.

Note: Wash windows when the sun isn't shining on them, which causes the mixture to dry too quickly and can result in streaks.

Natural Heavy-Duty Scrub

Ingredients

- 1/4 cup borax powder
- 4 Tablespoons lemon juice

Instructions

Mix the borax and lemon juice in a glass bowl to form a paste. It should be thick and slightly granular. Borax can be found at the grocery store in the laundry detergent aisle.

Suitable for:

- Cleaning tough spots on stove tops
- Water stains
- Discoloration stains

Natural Disinfectant

Ingredients

- 2 cups distilled water
- 1/3 cup vinegar
- 1 teaspoon sodium carbonate (washing soda)
- 10 to 15 drops of tea tree essential oil

Instructions

1. In a glass bowl, mix the ingredients until well combined.
2. Transfer to a glass jar or spray bottle and apply as needed.

Carpet Freshener and Deodorizer

Ingredients

- Baking Soda
- Essential oil

Instructions

1. Combine baking soda and enough essential oil in a bowl to give it a pleasant but not overbearing smell.
2. Sprinkle the mixture over a carpeted area and let it soak in for about an hour.
3. Once somewhat absorbed, ensure your vacuum is on the deepest carpet setting and vacuum it up.

Note: Any essential oil will work for this recipe as it is more for the scent than for a practical purpose. You do not need to use an oil if you prefer that it doesn't have a smell.

Peppermint Toilet Bombs

Ingredients

- 2 cups baking soda
- 1 cup citric acid
- 20 drops of tea tree essential oil
- 10 drops of lavender essential oil
- 10 drops of peppermint essential oil
- Approximately 3 tablespoons of white vinegar

Instructions

1. In a glass bowl, combine the baking soda and citric acid, stirring until fully combined.
2. In a separate bowl, combine the essential oils and stir well. Add more lavender if necessary if the smell doesn't pull through slightly.

3. Combine the ingredients from both bowls and mix well — it is very important that everything is very well stirred together at this point.
4. Then, add the white vinegar to a spray bottle and lightly spritz the mixture. Mix again and spritz for a second time. Repeat this process until the mixture can be shaped into one-inch balls or squares.
5. Create the balls or squares, placing them on parchment paper and allowing them to set for four to six hours.
6. Once they are dried, they can be stored in a container.
7. When using them, put one bomb in the toilet, and once it stops fizzing, use a toilet bowl brush to scrub the toilet and then flush it.

APPENDIX 1: GLOSSARY

Carcinogenic – a substance that may cause cancer.

Endocrine disrupter – a substance that has the ability to affect hormones.

Obesogen – a chemical or toxin that affects the metabolic system thereby causing weight gain.

Organic (when referring to toxins) – an toxin that contains the element carbon.

Organic (when not referring to toxins) – a product free from chemicals, toxins, hormones, antibiotics, etc.

APPENDIX 2: REPLACEMENT LIST

The following chart can be used to create a list of items around the home you wish to replace. I recommend starting with cleaners, personal care products, and items with a strong chemical smell.

Room	Replacement Items
Kitchen	
Dining room	
Bathroom	
Laundry room	
Living room	
Bedroom	
Groceries	

APPENDIX 3: SHOPPING FOR DETOX ITEMS

When purchasing products, especially those we use daily, it is essential to prioritize our health and well-being. With the increasing awareness about the harmful effects of toxins and chemicals in products, many consumers are now seeking out toxin-free alternatives. But where can you find these products?

Fortunately, several options are available for those looking to buy toxin-free products. One of the most convenient ways is to shop online. Many e-commerce platforms now have dedicated sections or filters specifically for eco-friendly and toxin-free products. This allows you to easily browse through a comprehensive range of options from the comfort of your own home.

Another option is to visit local health food stores or organic markets. These establishments often carry a variety of toxin-free products, ranging from personal care items to household cleaners and even clothing. Shopping at these stores ensures that you support local businesses and allows you to ask questions and receive personalized recommendations from knowledgeable staff.

APPENDIX 3: SHOPPING FOR DETOX ITEMS

Additionally, keep an eye out for certifications such as organic, natural, or non-toxic when shopping for products. These labels indicate that the product has undergone rigorous testing and meets specific ingredient quality and safety standards.

Finding toxic-free products is becoming more accessible as consumer demand grows. Whether you choose to shop online, visit local stores, look for certifications, or try your hand at DIY solutions, prioritizing your health by opting for non-toxic alternatives is a decision that benefits both you and the environment.

Some of my favorite brands and places to shop for organic, non-toxic products at the time of writing this book are listed below. Companies and products change over time, so always check the ingredients to ensure they haven't changed in a negative direction. You may find them to be excellent places to begin your wellness journey! Local farmer's markets are also a great place to find all-natural and organic products

Online Markets:

- **Azure Standard:** Contains thousands of household items that are organic and natural
- **Amazon:** Contains a wide range of products
- **Carina Organics:** Natural shampoos, conditioners, soaps, and baby wash items
- **iHerb:** Ships throughout the world, natural and organic items available. Check ingredients
- **Mountain Rose Herbs:** Organic herbs
- **New Directions Aromatics:** Raw ingredients for cosmetic making
- **Now Foods:** Organic essential oils

APPENDIX 3: SHOPPING FOR DETOX ITEMS

- **Thrive Market:** Contains many household products
- **Well.ca:** Has a Green section with items for throughout the home

Brands:

- **Attitude:** Cleaning and personal care products
- **Aunt Fannie's:** Cleaning products
- **BirchBabe:** Makeup and face cleaners
- **Branch Basics:** Household cleaners
- **Caboo:** Sustainable, chemical free bamboo toilet paper, paper towels and wipes
- **DivaCup:** Menstrual cups and discs
- **Dyson:** Air purifiers capable of removing formaldehyde and more
- **Extrema:** 100% ceramic cookware and bakeware
- **Hello:** Deodorant, toothpaste
- **Juice Beauty:** Organic and EWG certified beauty products
- **Lifestraw:** Water filters and purifiers
- **Meliora Cleaning Products:** Cleaning products
- **Nature Clean:** Dish soap, dish detergent, laundry detergent, toilet bowl cleaner, and more
- **NatraCare:** Plastic free, disposable pads
- **Schmidt's:** Deodorants
- **Saje Natural Wellness:** 100% natural aromatherapy products
- **Sapadilla Soap Company:** All-purpose cleaner concentrate, dish soap, laundry
- **Silk & Snow:** Reasonably priced better for you mattresses

APPENDIX 3: SHOPPING FOR DETOX ITEMS

- **Tanit:** Natural and plastic free cleaning products, toothpastes, personal care items and more

APPENDIX 4: DETOX CHECKLIST

The following list contains products that often contain toxins. Consider changing the following small items that can easily be exchanged for non-toxic alternatives. The following are easy and relatively easy swaps with no requirements for specific stores or trips.

Kitchen
- Plastic food storage containers
- Plastic cooking utensils
- Teflon cookware
- Pure aluminum cookware
- Plastic water bottles
- Dish soap/detergent
- Unfiltered water
- Cling film and aluminum foil
- Microwaves
- Cleaning solutions
- Junk food

Bathroom
- Toilet bowl cleaners
- Perfumes
- Multipurpose/surface cleaners
- Glass cleaner
- Shower curtains
- Bath mats
- Makeup
- Nail polish & remover
- Medications
- Deodorant
- Feminine hygiene products
- Diapers
- Toilet paper
- Hair dye

Bedroom
- Fast fashion
- Curtains
- Yoga mats

Livingroom
- Candles
- Plugins
- Air Freshener Sprays

Laundry room
- Laundry detergents
- Bleach
- Dryer sheets
- Stain removers
- Room sprays
- Floor cleaners

Office
- Correction fluid
- Receipts

Playroom
- Plastic toys

Garage & Outside
- Antifreeze
- Insecticides
- Pesticides
- Rat poison
- Fertilizers
- Car mats

Other
- E-cigarettes
- Some house plants
- Wifi

REFERENCES

Chapter 1
[1] Toxics Use Reduction in the Home: Lessons Learned from Household Exposure Studies by Sarah C. Dunagan,* Robin E. Dodson, Ruthann A. Rudel, and Julia G. Brody
[2] *Microplastics Have Been Found In The Human Bloodstream.* (n.d.). Henry Ford Health - Detroit, MI. https://www.henryford.com/blog/2022/04/microplastics-in-human-bloodstream
[3] Afkr. (2019, June 24). *Plastic ingestion by people could be equating to a credit card a week.* The University of Newcastle, Australia. https://www.newcastle.edu.au/newsroom/featured/plastic-ingestion-by-people-could-be-equating-to-a-credit-card-a-week
[4] Chemical Safety and Health Unit. (2016). The public health impact of chemicals: knowns and unknowns. *www.who.int.* https://www.who.int/publications/i/item/WHO-FWC-PHE-EPE-16-01
[5] Yates, D. (n.d.). *Environmental contaminants alter gut microbiome, health.* https://news.illinois.edu/view/6367/808857
[6] *Bisphenol A (BPA).* (2023, August 31). National Institute of Environmental Health Sciences. https://www.niehs.nih.gov/health/topics/agents/sya-bpa/index.cfm
[7] Thoene, M., Dzika, E., Gonkowski, S., & Wojtkiewicz, J. (2020). Bisphenol S in Food Causes Hormonal and Obesogenic Effects Comparable to or Worse than Bisphenol A: A Literature Review. *Nutrients, 12*(2), 532. https://doi.org/10.3390/nu12020532
[8] Thoene, M., Dzika, E., Gonkowski, S., & Wojtkiewicz, J. (2020b). Bisphenol S in Food Causes Hormonal and Obesogenic Effects Comparable to or Worse than Bisphenol A: A Literature Review. *Nutrients, 12*(2), 532. https://doi.org/10.3390/nu12020532
[9] Toxic-Free Future. (2022, September 20). *Additional quotes - Toxic-Free Future.* https://toxicfreefuture.org/mind-the-store/rei-ban-pfas/additional-quotes/

Chapter 2
[1] *Endocrine Disruptors.* (2023, June 2). National Institute of Environmental Health Sciences. https://www.niehs.nih.gov/health/topics/agents/endocrine/index.cfm
[2] Society, E. (2019). Impact of EDCs on reproductive systems. *Endocrine*

REFERENCES

Society. https://www.endocrine.org/topics/edc/what-edcs-are/common-edcs/reproduction

[3] Society, E. (2019b). Impact of EDCs on reproductive systems. *Endocrine Society.* https://www.endocrine.org/topics/edc/what-edcs-are/common-edcs/reproduction

[4] Dunagan, S. C., Dodson, R. E., Rudel, R. A., & Brody, J. G. (2011). Toxics use reduction in the home: lessons learned from household exposure studies. *Journal of Cleaner Production, 19*(5), 438–444. https://doi.org/10.1016/j.jclepro.2010.06.012

[5] Tu, P., Chi, L., Bodnar, W. M., Zhang, Z., Gao, B., Bian, X., Stewart, J. R., Fry, R. C., & Lü, K. (2020). Gut Microbiome toxicity: Connecting the environment and Gut Microbiome-Associated diseases. *Toxics, 8*(1), 19. https://doi.org/10.3390/toxics8010019

[6] Suzy Kassem, Rise Up and Salute the Sun: The Writings of Suzy Kassem

[7] The scientific article, 'Toxicology of food dyes' states the following concerns with food dyes:

- Red 3: causes cancer in animals
- Red 40: contaminated with benzidine or other carcinogens; causes hypersensitivity reactions
- Yellow 5: contaminated with benzidine or other carcinogens; causes hypersensitivity reactions
- Yellow 6: contaminated with benzidine or other carcinogens; causes hypersensitivity reactions
- Blue 1: causes hypersensitivity reactions

Kobylewski, S., & Jacobson, M. F. (2012). Toxicology of food dyes. *International Journal of Occupational and Environmental Health, 18*(3), 220–246. https://doi.org/10.1179/1077352512z.00000000034

[8] *What is BPA? Should I be worried about it?* (2023, March 24). Mayo Clinic. https://www.mayoclinic.org/healthy-lifestyle/nutrition-and-healthy-eating/expert-answers/bpa/faq-20058331

Chapter 3

[1] Holden, E. (2021, October 22). Is modern life poisoning me? I took the tests to find out. *The Guardian.*https://www.theguardian.com/us-news/2019/may/22/is-modern-life-poisoning-me-i-took-the-tests-to-find-out

[2] Rather than keep referring you back to chapter one for more information about a specific chemical or toxin, I have noted this with an asterisk (*).

REFERENCES

Therefore, when you see the symbol, know that when you need more information (or just a refresher) about it, please jump back to chapter one.

[3] Example of a label.

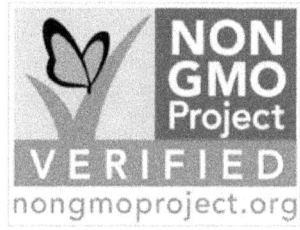

Chapter 4

[1] Rather than keep referring you back to chapter one for more information about a specific chemical or toxin, I have noted this with an asterisk (*). Therefore, when you see the symbol, know that when you need more information (or just a refresher) about it, please jump back to chapter one.

[2] Benzoni, T. (2023, June 26). *Bleach toxicity*. StatPearls - NCBI Bookshelf. https://www.ncbi.nlm.nih.gov/books/NBK441921/

[3] Lin, N., Ding, N., Meza-Wilson, E., Devasurendra, A. M., Godwin, C., Park, S. K., & Batterman, S. (2020). Volatile organic compounds in feminine hygiene products sold in the US market: A survey of products and health risks. *Environment International, 144*, 105740. https://doi.org/10.1016/j.envint.2020.105740

[4] Reference: Guenard, R. (2015, January 2). Hair Dye: a History. *The Atlantic*. https://www.theatlantic.com/health/archive/2015/01/hair-dye-a-history/383934/

[5] Heikkinen, S., Pitkäniemi, J., Sarkeala, T., Malila, N., & Koskenvuo, M. (2015). Does hair dye use increase the risk of breast cancer? A Population-Based Case-Control Study of Finnish women. *PLOS ONE, 10*(8), e0135190. https://doi.org/10.1371/journal.pone.0135190

Chapter 6

[1] *Potentially harmful chemicals found in plastic toys*. (2021, February 21). ScienceDaily. https://www.sciencedaily.com/releases/2021/02/210222124552.htm

Chapter 7

[1] *What is radon gas? Is it dangerous? | US EPA*. (2022, October 24). US EPA. https://www.epa.gov/radiation/what-radon-gas-it-dangerous

[2] *Dangers of chlorine? - ask Dr. Weil*. (2016, December 4). DrWeil.com. https://www.drweil.com/health-wellness/balanced-living/healthy-living/dangers-of-chlorine/

REFERENCES

Chapter 8

[1] *Meet Generation Z: Shaping the future of shopping.* (2020, August 4). McKinsey & Company. https://www.mckinsey.com/industries/consumer-packaged-goods/our-insights/meet-generation-z-shaping-the-future-of-shopping

[2] Goldberg, S. (2022). Lithium mining: dirty investment or sustainable business? *Investopedia.* https://www.investopedia.com/investing/lithium-mining-dirty-investment-or-sustainable-business/

[3] Eagleman, D. (2010). *Incognito: The Secret Lives of the Brain.* Viking.

www.ingramcontent.com/pod-product-compliance
Lightning Source LLC
Chambersburg PA
CBHW070043040426
42333CB00041B/2176